NON-PHARMACEUTICAL INTERVENTIONS FOR NAUSEA AND VOMITING IN PREGNANCY:

USING DIET, EXERCISE, AROMATHERAPY, AND OTHER NATURAL REMEDIES TO MANAGE MORNING SICKNESS

BY

HENRY E. PARKINS

COPYRIGHT PAGE

TABLE OF CONTENTS

COPYRIGHT PAGE   2

TABLE OF CONTENTS   3

INTRODUCTION   8

**Definition and Significance of Nausea and Vomiting in Pregnancy
(NVP)**   11

**Importance of Non-Pharmaceutical Interventions (NPIs) in Managing
Nausea and Vomiting in Pregnancy (NVP)**   14

**Overview of the Book: "Non-Pharmaceutical Interventions for
Nausea and Vomiting in Pregnancy"**   17

CHAPTER 1   22

UNDERSTANDING NAUSEA AND VOMITING IN PREGNANCY
(NVP)   22

**Causes and Contributing Factors of Nausea and Vomiting in
Pregnancy (NVP)**   25

Impact on Maternal Health and Quality of Life   28

Potential Risks to Fetal Well-being   31

CHAPTER 2   35

NON-PHARMACEUTICAL INTERVENTIONS (NPIS): AN
OVERVIEW   35

Definition and Scope of Non-Pharmaceutical Interventions (NPIs)   38

Types of Non-Pharmaceutical Interventions (NPIs) Commonly Used for Managing Nausea and Vomiting in Pregnancy (NVP)   42

Evidence-Based Practices and Guidelines for Non-Pharmaceutical Interventions (NPIs)   45

CHAPTER 3   48

DIETARY MODIFICATIONS AND NUTRITIONAL STRATEGIES   48

The Importance of Diet in Managing Nausea and Vomiting in Pregnancy (NVP)   52

Dietary Modifications for Alleviating NVP Symptoms   55

Specific Dietary Modifications to Alleviate Symptoms   57

Nutritional Supplements in NVP Management   59

CHAPTER 4   63

LIFESTYLE MODIFICATIONS AND BEHAVIORAL STRATEGIES FOR NVP MANAGEMENT   63

Stress Reduction Techniques for NVP Management   67

Relaxation Exercises and Mindfulness Practices   70

Relaxation Exercises and Mindfulness Practices for Nausea and Vomiting in Pregnancy   73

CHAPTER 5   76

SLEEP HYGIENE AND ITS IMPACT ON NAUSEA AND VOMITING IN PREGNANCY (NVP)   76

Alternative Therapies and Complementary Medicine for Nausea and Vomiting in Pregnancy   80

Acupressure and Acupuncture: Alternative Therapies for Nausea and Vomiting in Pregnancy   82

Herbal Remedies and Aromatherapy for Managing Nausea and Vomiting in Pregnancy   86

Yoga and Mind-Body Interventions for Managing Nausea and Vomiting in Pregnancy   89

CHAPTER 6   93

SUPPORTIVE CARE AND PRACTICAL TIPS FOR MANAGING NAUSEA AND VOMITING IN PREGNANCY   93

Emotional Support for Pregnant Individuals Experiencing Nausea and Vomiting in Pregnancy (NVP)   96

Practical Tips for Managing Nausea and Vomiting in Pregnancy (NVP) at Home and Work   100

Importance of Communication with Healthcare Providers   103

CHAPTER 7   107

EVALUATING EFFECTIVENESS AND SAFETY OF NON-PHARMACEUTICAL INTERVENTIONS (NPIS)   107

Methods for Assessing the Effectiveness of Non-Pharmaceutical Interventions (NPIs) in Managing Nausea and Vomiting in Pregnancy (NVP)   110

Safety Considerations and Potential Risks of Non-Pharmaceutical Interventions (NPIs)   113

Monitoring and Adjusting Interventions Based on Individual Needs   117

CHAPTER 8   121

INTEGRATIVE APPROACHES TO NVP MANAGEMENT   121

Combining Multiple NPIs for Enhanced Symptom Relief   124

Integrating NPIs with Pharmacological Interventions When Necessary   127

Holistic Approaches to Promoting Overall Maternal Well-being   131

CHAPTER 9   134

FUTURE DIRECTIONS AND RESEARCH OPPORTUNITIES   134

Emerging Trends in NPIs for NVP Management   138

Areas for Further Research and Innovation   142

Potential Implications for Clinical Practice and Public Health Policy   146

CHAPTER 11   149

CONCLUSION   149

Summary of Key Findings and Insights: 151

Final Thoughts on the Future of NPIs in Improving Maternal and Fetal Health   157

INTRODUCTION

Nausea and vomiting in pregnancy (NVP), often colloquially known as "morning sickness," are among the most common and challenging symptoms experienced by pregnant individuals worldwide. While NVP is typically considered a normal part of pregnancy, its severity and impact can vary widely among individuals, ranging from mild discomfort to debilitating symptoms that significantly affect daily functioning and quality of life.

In recent years, there has been growing recognition of the limitations and potential risks associated with pharmaceutical interventions for managing NVP, particularly in light of concerns about fetal safety and long-term health outcomes. As a result, there has been increasing interest in exploring non-pharmaceutical interventions (NPIs) as safe and effective alternatives for alleviating NVP symptoms and improving maternal well-being.

This book, "Non-Pharmaceutical Interventions for Nausea and Vomiting in Pregnancy," is a comprehensive exploration of evidence-based strategies and approaches for managing NVP without the use of traditional medications. Drawing upon the latest research and clinical insights, this book aims to provide healthcare professionals, expectant mothers, and their families with practical guidance and support in navigating the challenges of NVP.

At its core, this book is founded on the principle of holistic care, recognizing the interconnectedness of physical, emotional, and environmental factors in influencing the experience of NVP. By taking a multidimensional approach to NVP management, we aim to empower individuals with a diverse toolkit of strategies and interventions tailored to their unique needs and preferences.

Throughout the chapters that follow, readers will find a wealth of information on dietary modifications, lifestyle changes, alternative therapies, and supportive care techniques that have shown promise in relieving NVP symptoms and promoting maternal well-being. From simple dietary adjustments to more complex integrative approaches, each intervention is carefully examined in terms of its evidence base,

8

safety profile, and practical application in real-world settings.

Importantly, this book also seeks to foster a deeper understanding of the psychosocial and emotional dimensions of NVP, acknowledging the profound impact that these symptoms can have on an individual's mental health, self-esteem, and sense of identity as a parent-to-be. By addressing the emotional needs of pregnant individuals with compassion and empathy, we hope to create a supportive environment where individuals feel empowered to seek help and advocate for their own well-being.

As we embark on this journey together, it is our sincere hope that this book will serve as a valuable resource for healthcare providers, researchers, educators, and anyone who shares a passion for improving the lives of pregnant individuals and their families. By embracing a collaborative and patient-centered approach to NVP management, we can work together to ensure that every pregnancy is characterized by comfort, support, and the opportunity for joyous anticipation of new life.

Definition and Significance of Nausea and Vomiting in Pregnancy (NVP)

Nausea and vomiting in pregnancy (NVP), commonly referred to as "morning sickness," encompass a range of symptoms experienced by pregnant individuals, typically during the first trimester of pregnancy. While the term "morning sickness" implies that symptoms are confined to the morning hours, many individuals experience NVP throughout the day and night, with varying degrees of severity.

NVP is characterized by feelings of nausea, often accompanied by episodes of vomiting or retching. These symptoms can range from mild and occasional discomfort to severe and persistent nausea that significantly impairs daily functioning and quality of life. In some cases, NVP can progress to a more severe form known as hyperemesis gravidarum, characterized by excessive vomiting, dehydration, and electrolyte imbalances requiring medical intervention.

The significance of NVP extends beyond its physical manifestations, encompassing a wide range of psychosocial, emotional, and practical implications for pregnant individuals and their families. For many expectant mothers, NVP can be a source of considerable distress, anxiety, and frustration, disrupting normal routines, interfering with work or social activities, and undermining feelings of well-being and confidence during pregnancy.

Moreover, NVP can have profound implications for maternal and fetal health, particularly when symptoms are severe and prolonged. Persistent vomiting and inadequate nutrition can lead to dehydration, electrolyte imbalances, weight loss, and nutritional deficiencies, potentially compromising maternal health and fetal development. In cases of hyperemesis gravidarum, there is an increased risk of complications such as preterm birth, low birth weight, and maternal hospitalization.

Beyond the immediate health concerns, NVP can also have long-lasting effects on maternal mental health and well-being. The psychological toll of coping with chronic nausea and vomiting, coupled with the uncertainty and unpredictability of symptoms, can contribute to feelings of isolation, depression, and anxiety. For some individuals, NVP may evoke fears and anxieties about the health and viability of the pregnancy, further exacerbating emotional distress.

Given the prevalence and impact of NVP on pregnant individuals and their families, effective management strategies are essential to mitigate symptoms, alleviate distress, and promote maternal and fetal well-being. While pharmaceutical interventions have traditionally been used to manage NVP, there is growing recognition of the limitations and potential risks associated with these medications, particularly in light of concerns about fetal safety and long-term health outcomes.

In this context, non-pharmaceutical interventions (NPIs) offer a promising alternative for managing NVP, providing safe, effective, and evidence-based strategies to alleviate symptoms and improve quality of life for pregnant individuals. By addressing the multidimensional nature of NVP and considering the unique needs and preferences of each individual, NPIs hold the potential to empower pregnant individuals with a diverse toolkit of interventions tailored to their specific circumstances.

Importance of Non-Pharmaceutical Interventions (NPIs) in Managing Nausea and Vomiting in Pregnancy (NVP)

Non-pharmaceutical interventions (NPIs) play a pivotal role in the comprehensive management of nausea and vomiting in pregnancy (NVP), offering safe, effective, and holistic strategies to alleviate symptoms, improve maternal well-being, and optimize fetal outcomes. While pharmaceutical treatments have traditionally been used to manage NVP, the importance of NPIs lies in their ability to provide alternative approaches that minimize potential risks and promote overall health and wellness for pregnant individuals.

Safety and Minimal Risk: NPIs offer a range of interventions that are generally considered safe for use during pregnancy, minimizing the potential risks associated with pharmacological treatments. By focusing on natural and non-invasive approaches, NPIs prioritize maternal and fetal safety, providing peace of mind for expectant mothers and healthcare providers alike.

Patient-Centered Care: NPIs emphasize a patient-centered approach to NVP management, recognizing the unique needs, preferences, and experiences of each individual. By empowering pregnant individuals to actively participate in their care and decision-making process, NPIs foster a sense of autonomy, control, and empowerment, enhancing overall satisfaction with the treatment process.

Comprehensive Symptom Management: NPIs encompass a diverse array of interventions that target the multidimensional nature of NVP, addressing not only physical symptoms but also psychosocial and emotional factors that contribute to distress and discomfort.

From dietary modifications and lifestyle changes to alternative therapies and supportive care techniques, NPIs provide a comprehensive toolkit for symptom management that can be tailored to the individual needs of each patient.

Minimal Environmental Impact:

Many NPIs are environmentally friendly and sustainable, minimizing the use of pharmaceuticals and reducing the environmental footprint associated with healthcare delivery. By promoting natural and eco-friendly interventions, NPIs align with principles of environmental stewardship and sustainability, contributing to broader efforts to protect and preserve the planet for future generations.

Empowerment and Self-Care:

NPIs empower pregnant individuals with practical skills, knowledge, and resources to actively manage their symptoms and promote their own well-being. By incorporating self-care practices into daily routines, such as mindfulness techniques, relaxation exercises, and dietary modifications, NPIs foster a sense of self-efficacy and resilience, enabling individuals to navigate the challenges of NVP with confidence and optimism.

Cost-Effective and Accessible:

Many NPIs are cost-effective and accessible, making them suitable for individuals with diverse socioeconomic backgrounds and resource constraints. By leveraging simple and affordable interventions, such as dietary modifications and home-based therapies, NPIs ensure equitable access to care and support for pregnant individuals across different settings and communities.

Overview of the Book: "Non-Pharmaceutical Interventions for Nausea and Vomiting in Pregnancy"

The book "Non-Pharmaceutical Interventions for Nausea and Vomiting in Pregnancy" serves as a comprehensive resource for healthcare professionals, expectant mothers, and their families seeking safe, effective, and holistic strategies for managing nausea and vomiting during pregnancy (NVP). Rooted in evidence-based practices and clinical insights, this book aims to provide a thorough exploration of non-pharmaceutical interventions (NPIs) while addressing the multifaceted challenges posed by NVP.

Objectives:

Provide a Comprehensive Understanding: The book aims to deepen the reader's understanding of NVP by examining its causes, risk factors, and impact on maternal and fetal health. By elucidating the complex nature of NVP, readers gain insights into the diverse manifestations and underlying mechanisms of this common pregnancy symptom.

Explore Evidence-Based NPIs: Through a rigorous review of the latest research and clinical evidence, the book identifies and evaluates a range of non-pharmaceutical interventions for managing NVP. From dietary modifications and lifestyle changes to alternative therapies and supportive care techniques, readers gain practical insights into effective strategies for alleviating symptoms and enhancing maternal well-being.

Foster a Holistic Approach: Recognizing the interconnectedness of physical, emotional, and environmental factors in shaping the experience of NVP, the book emphasizes a holistic approach to NVP management. By integrating diverse interventions that address the whole person, readers learn how to tailor care plans to meet the unique needs and preferences of each individual.

Empower Patients and Providers: By equipping readers with knowledge, skills, and resources, the book empowers both patients and healthcare providers to actively engage in the management of NVP. Through practical guidance and actionable recommendations, readers learn how to collaborate effectively, make informed decisions, and optimize outcomes for pregnant individuals and their families.

Structure:

Introduction: The book begins with an overview of NVP, its significance, and the rationale for exploring non-pharmaceutical interventions as alternative approaches to management.

Understanding NVP: This section delves into the causes, risk factors, and physiological mechanisms underlying NVP, providing readers with a foundational understanding of this common pregnancy symptom.

Non-Pharmaceutical Interventions (NPIs): An Overview: Readers are introduced to the concept of NPIs and the diverse range of interventions available for managing NVP.

Dietary Modifications and Nutritional Strategies: This section explores the role of diet and nutrition in NVP management, highlighting evidence-based dietary modifications and nutritional supplements.

Lifestyle Modifications and Behavioral Strategies: Readers learn about lifestyle changes, stress reduction techniques, and behavioral strategies that can help alleviate NVP symptoms and improve maternal well-being.

Alternative Therapies and Complementary Medicine: The book examines alternative therapies such as acupuncture, acupressure, herbal remedies, and aromatherapy, exploring their potential efficacy and safety in NVP management.

Supportive Care and Practical Tips: Practical guidance and supportive care techniques are provided for pregnant individuals and their families, including emotional support, coping strategies, and practical tips for symptom relief.

Evaluating Effectiveness and Safety of NPIs: This section discusses methods for evaluating the effectiveness and safety of NPIs, empowering readers to make informed decisions about their care.

Integrative Approaches to NVP Management: Readers learn how to integrate multiple NPIs into comprehensive care plans, maximizing symptom relief and promoting overall maternal and fetal well-being.

Future Directions and Research Opportunities: The book concludes with a discussion of emerging trends, research opportunities, and implications for clinical practice and public health policy.

Through its comprehensive objectives and structured approach, "Non-Pharmaceutical Interventions for Nausea and Vomiting in Pregnancy" aims to empower readers with the knowledge, skills, and confidence to effectively manage NVP and optimize outcomes for pregnant individuals and their families.

CHAPTER 1

UNDERSTANDING NAUSEA AND VOMITING IN PREGNANCY (NVP)

Nausea and vomiting in pregnancy (NVP), commonly known as "morning sickness," represent a complex and multifaceted phenomenon that affects a significant proportion of pregnant individuals worldwide. While NVP is often considered a normal part of pregnancy, its impact can vary widely in terms of severity, duration, and associated distress.

Causes and Contributing Factors:

NVP is thought to result from a combination of hormonal, physiological, and psychological factors. The rise in hormone levels, particularly human chorionic gonadotropin (hCG) and estrogen, during early pregnancy is believed to play a central role in triggering NVP symptoms. Other contributing factors may include changes in gastrointestinal motility, alterations in sensory perception, genetic predisposition, and psychosocial stressors.

Timing and Duration: NVP typically manifests during the first trimester of pregnancy, with symptoms peaking around 9-10 weeks gestation and gradually subsiding by the end of the first trimester for most individuals. However, some pregnant individuals may experience NVP throughout pregnancy, while others may have symptoms that persist beyond the first trimester, requiring ongoing management and support.

Severity and Impact: While NVP is commonly perceived as a minor inconvenience, it can have a significant impact on the physical, emotional, and social well-being of pregnant individuals. For many, NVP symptoms can be debilitating, interfering with daily activities, work responsibilities, and social engagements. Severe and persistent NVP, such as hyperemesis gravidarum, can lead to dehydration, electrolyte imbalances, weight loss, and psychological distress, posing risks to maternal and fetal health.

Risk Factors and Vulnerable Populations: Certain factors may increase the likelihood of experiencing NVP or developing more severe symptoms. These risk factors may include a history of NVP in previous pregnancies, multiple gestations (e.g., twins or higher-order multiples), young maternal age, first-time pregnancy, and pre-existing gastrointestinal conditions. Additionally, there is evidence to suggest that socioeconomic factors, stress, and lifestyle habits may influence the onset and severity of NVP symptoms.

Impact on Maternal-Fetal Health: While NVP is generally considered a benign condition, severe and prolonged symptoms may pose risks to maternal and fetal health. Persistent vomiting and inadequate nutrition can lead to dehydration, electrolyte imbalances, nutritional deficiencies, and maternal weight loss. In severe cases, maternal hospitalization may be necessary to manage complications and ensure the well-being of both mother and baby. Additionally, there is evidence to suggest that maternal stress and anxiety associated with NVP may impact fetal development and contribute to adverse pregnancy outcomes.

Causes and Contributing Factors of Nausea and Vomiting in Pregnancy (NVP)

Nausea and vomiting in pregnancy (NVP) is a common and often distressing symptom experienced by many pregnant individuals. While the exact etiology of NVP remains elusive, several factors are believed to contribute to its onset and severity. Understanding these causes and contributing factors is essential for implementing effective non-pharmaceutical interventions (NPIs) to manage NVP. Here are key considerations:

Hormonal Changes:

Hormonal fluctuations, particularly an increase in circulating levels of human chorionic gonadotropin (hCG) and estrogen, are widely implicated in the pathophysiology of NVP. These hormonal changes occur rapidly during early pregnancy and are believed to stimulate the chemoreceptor trigger zone (CTZ) in the brain, leading to nausea and vomiting.

Gastrointestinal Changes:

Pregnancy is associated with various physiological changes in the gastrointestinal (GI) tract, including alterations in gastric motility, delayed gastric emptying, and relaxation of the lower esophageal sphincter. These changes can contribute to symptoms of nausea and vomiting by increasing gastric distension and delaying the clearance of gastric contents.

Sensory and Psychological Factors:

Sensory hypersensitivity to odors, tastes, and visual stimuli is common in pregnancy and may exacerbate symptoms of nausea and vomiting. Additionally, psychological factors such as anxiety, stress, and emotional distress have been implicated in the severity and duration of NVP. The psychosocial context of pregnancy, including social support, socioeconomic status, and cultural beliefs, may also influence the perception and management of NVP.

Genetic Predisposition: There is evidence to suggest that genetic factors may play a role in predisposing individuals to NVP. Family history of NVP, particularly in first-degree relatives, has been associated with an increased risk of experiencing severe symptoms. Twin and sibling studies further support the hereditary component of NVP, although specific genetic markers have yet to be identified.

Trophoblastic Theory: The trophoblastic theory posits that NVP may serve an adaptive function in pregnancy by protecting the developing embryo from potentially harmful substances and pathogens. According to this theory, the aversion to certain foods and smells, as well as the act of vomiting, may help prevent maternal exposure to toxins and pathogens during a critical period of embryonic development.

Environmental and Lifestyle Factors: Environmental exposures, such as air pollution, occupational hazards, and dietary factors, may contribute to the onset or exacerbation of NVP symptoms.

Lifestyle factors, including smoking, alcohol consumption, and dietary habits, have also been implicated in the severity of NVP. Additionally, pre-existing gastrointestinal conditions, such as gastroesophageal reflux disease (GERD) and irritable bowel syndrome (IBS), may increase the risk of experiencing more severe NVP symptoms.

Impact on Maternal Health and Quality of Life

Nausea and vomiting in pregnancy (NVP) can have a profound impact on the physical, emotional, and social well-being of pregnant individuals, often affecting their overall quality of life and maternal health. Understanding the far-reaching consequences of NVP is crucial for implementing effective non-pharmaceutical interventions (NPIs) to mitigate its impact and improve maternal outcomes. Here are key considerations regarding the impact of NVP on maternal health and quality of life:

Nutritional Deficiencies and Weight Loss: Severe and persistent NVP symptoms can lead to inadequate nutrition, dehydration, and weight loss in pregnant individuals. The inability to tolerate food and fluids may result in nutritional deficiencies, including deficiencies in essential vitamins and minerals such as vitamin B6, vitamin B12, and folate, which are critical for maternal and fetal health.

Dehydration and Electrolyte Imbalance:
Excessive vomiting and fluid loss associated with NVP can lead to dehydration and electrolyte imbalances, posing risks to maternal health and fetal development. Electrolyte imbalances, such as hypokalemia and hyponatremia, can disrupt normal physiological processes and increase the risk of complications such as muscle cramps, fatigue, and cardiac arrhythmias.

Impact on Maternal Mental Health:
The chronicity and severity of NVP symptoms can significantly impact maternal mental health and emotional well-being. Pregnant individuals experiencing severe NVP may feel overwhelmed, anxious, and depressed, affecting their ability to cope with daily stressors and

engage in social activities. Persistent feelings of distress and isolation may exacerbate existing mental health conditions or lead to the development of perinatal mood disorders such as depression and anxiety.

Disruption of Daily Activities and Productivity: Severe NVP symptoms can disrupt daily activities, work responsibilities, and social engagements, diminishing maternal productivity and functional capacity. Pregnant individuals may struggle to maintain employment, attend to household duties, and care for other children or family members, leading to feelings of frustration, guilt, and inadequacy.

Impact on Maternal-Fetal Bonding and Pregnancy Experience: NVP can influence the maternal-fetal bond and shape the overall pregnancy experience for expectant mothers. The physical discomfort and emotional distress associated with NVP may detract from the joy and excitement of pregnancy, impacting the expectant

mother's ability to connect with her unborn baby and embrace the transformative journey of motherhood.

Healthcare Utilization and Economic Burden:
Severe NVP symptoms may necessitate frequent healthcare visits, emergency room visits, and hospitalizations for hydration and symptom management. The economic burden associated with healthcare utilization, medication costs, and lost productivity can place significant financial strain on pregnant individuals and their families, exacerbating socioeconomic disparities and barriers to care.

Potential Risks to Fetal Well-being

Nausea and vomiting in pregnancy (NVP), while primarily affecting the pregnant individual, can also have implications for fetal well-being, particularly when symptoms are severe and persistent. Understanding the potential risks to fetal health associated with NVP is essential for healthcare providers and expectant mothers alike. Here are key considerations regarding potential risks to fetal well-being:

Inadequate Nutritional Intake:

Severe and prolonged NVP symptoms can result in inadequate maternal nutrition, depriving the developing fetus of essential nutrients critical for growth and development. Insufficient intake of macronutrients, vitamins, and minerals may compromise fetal nutritional status, leading to impaired organ development, low birth weight, and other adverse perinatal outcomes.

Electrolyte Imbalance:

Excessive vomiting and fluid loss associated with NVP can lead to electrolyte imbalances in the pregnant individual, which may indirectly impact fetal well-being. Electrolyte disturbances, such as hypokalemia and hyponatremia, can disrupt normal fetal physiology and increase the risk of complications such as fetal distress, preterm birth, and intrauterine growth restriction (IUGR).

Maternal Dehydration:

Dehydration resulting from severe NVP symptoms can compromise maternal hemodynamic stability and placental perfusion, potentially compromising fetal oxygenation and nutrient delivery. Maternal dehydration may increase the risk of fetal hypoxia, acidosis, and placental insufficiency, which are associated with adverse fetal outcomes such as fetal distress, meconium aspiration, and stillbirth.

Medication Exposure: In cases where pharmacological interventions are required to manage severe NVP symptoms, there may be concerns regarding potential fetal exposure to medications. While certain antiemetic medications are considered safe for use during pregnancy, others may pose risks to fetal development and long-term health outcomes. Healthcare providers must weigh the benefits and risks of medication use in pregnancy and consider alternative non-pharmaceutical interventions when appropriate.

Impact on Fetal Growth and Development: Maternal stress, anxiety, and nutritional deficiencies associated with severe NVP symptoms may impact fetal growth and development during critical periods of embryogenesis and fetal

organogenesis. Poor maternal nutritional status and inadequate intrauterine nutrition may predispose the fetus to long-term metabolic, cardiovascular, and neurodevelopmental disorders later in life.

Psychological and Emotional Factors:

Maternal stress, depression, and emotional distress resulting from severe NVP symptoms can influence fetal neurodevelopment and the maternal-fetal bonding process. Prenatal exposure to maternal anxiety and depression has been linked to alterations in fetal neuroendocrine function, stress reactivity, and behavioral outcomes in childhood and adolescence.

Increased Risk of Preterm Birth and Low Birth Weight:

Severe NVP symptoms, particularly when associated with complications such as dehydration and electrolyte imbalances, may increase the risk of preterm birth and low birth weight. Preterm birth and low birth weight are significant risk factors for neonatal morbidity and mortality, as well as long-term developmental delays and health problems.

34

CHAPTER 2

NON-PHARMACEUTICAL INTERVENTIONS (NPIS): AN OVERVIEW

Non-pharmaceutical interventions (NPIs) represent a diverse array of strategies and approaches aimed at alleviating nausea and vomiting in pregnancy (NVP) without the use of traditional medications. As awareness of the limitations and potential risks associated with pharmaceutical treatments for NVP continues to grow, there has been increasing interest in exploring alternative approaches that prioritize safety, effectiveness, and patient-centered care. In this section, we provide an overview of key non-pharmaceutical interventions that have shown promise in managing NVP:

Dietary Modifications: Dietary modifications play a central role in NVP management, offering pregnant individuals opportunities to identify and avoid triggers that exacerbate symptoms. Recommendations may include consuming small, frequent meals to prevent gastric distension, avoiding spicy or fatty foods that may exacerbate nausea, and incorporating bland, easily digestible foods such as crackers, toast, and rice.

Hydration Strategies:

Adequate hydration is essential for managing NVP and preventing dehydration associated with excessive vomiting. Pregnant individuals are encouraged to sip fluids throughout the day, opting for clear liquids such as water, herbal teas, and electrolyte-rich beverages to replenish fluids and electrolytes lost through vomiting.

Acupressure and Acupuncture:

Acupressure and acupuncture are traditional Chinese medicine techniques that involve applying pressure or inserting needles into specific points on the body to alleviate nausea and vomiting. Research suggests that stimulating acupressure points, such as the P6 or Neiguan point on the inner wrist, may help reduce NVP symptoms and improve overall well-being.

Ginger Supplementation:

Ginger, a natural remedy with anti-nausea properties, has been studied for its potential efficacy in managing NVP. Pregnant individuals may consider incorporating ginger supplements, ginger tea, or ginger candies into their daily routine to help alleviate symptoms. However, it is important to consult with a healthcare provider before using ginger supplements, particularly at higher doses.

Aromatherapy: Aromatherapy involves the use of essential oils derived from plant extracts to promote relaxation and alleviate symptoms of nausea. Certain essential oils, such as peppermint, lemon, and lavender, may be diffused, diluted, or applied topically to help soothe NVP symptoms and enhance overall well-being. Pregnant individuals should exercise caution when using essential oils and consult with a qualified aromatherapist or healthcare provider.

Mindfulness and Relaxation Techniques: Mindfulness-based stress reduction techniques, relaxation exercises, and deep breathing techniques can help pregnant individuals manage stress, anxiety, and nausea associated with NVP. Practices such as yoga, meditation, guided imagery, and progressive muscle relaxation may promote a sense of calm, balance, and resilience during pregnancy.

Supportive Care and Peer Support: Emotional support from partners, family members, friends, and healthcare providers is invaluable for pregnant individuals experiencing NVP. Peer support groups, online forums, and community-based resources offer opportunities for pregnant individuals to connect with others facing similar challenges, share experiences, and access practical tips and coping strategies.

Definition and Scope of Non-Pharmaceutical Interventions (NPIs)

Non-pharmaceutical interventions (NPIs) encompass a wide range of strategies and approaches aimed at alleviating nausea and vomiting in pregnancy (NVP) without the use of traditional medications. In the context of managing NVP, NPIs prioritize safety, effectiveness, and patient-centered care, offering pregnant individuals alternative options for symptom relief and improved quality of life. The definition and scope of NPIs within the context of NVP management include the following components:

Holistic Approach: NPIs embrace a holistic approach to NVP management, recognizing the interconnectedness of physical, emotional, and environmental factors that contribute to symptoms. By addressing the whole person, NPIs strive to promote overall well-being and enhance the pregnancy experience for expectant mothers.

Multimodal Strategies: NPIs encompass a diverse array of interventions that target various aspects of NVP, including dietary modifications, lifestyle changes, alternative therapies, supportive care techniques, and psychosocial interventions. The scope of NPIs extends beyond individual interventions to encompass integrated care plans tailored to meet the unique needs and preferences of each pregnant individual.

Evidence-Based Practices: NPIs are grounded in evidence-based practices and clinical guidelines supported by scientific research and clinical expertise.

While the evidence base for some NPIs may vary in terms of quality and strength, efforts are made to prioritize interventions with demonstrated efficacy, safety, and feasibility in the management of NVP.

Safety and Risk Mitigation: Safety considerations are paramount in the selection and implementation of NPIs for NVP management. Pregnant individuals and healthcare providers collaborate to identify interventions that pose minimal risk to maternal and fetal health, taking into account potential contraindications, adverse effects, and safety profiles associated with certain modalities.

Patient-Centered Care: NPIs emphasize a patient-centered approach to NVP management, empowering pregnant individuals to actively participate in decision-making processes, goal setting, and treatment planning. The scope of NPIs extends beyond symptom relief to address the emotional, psychosocial, and practical needs of pregnant individuals throughout the pregnancy journey.

Complementary to Pharmacological Interventions:

While NPIs offer alternative options for managing NVP, they are complementary to pharmacological interventions and may be used alone or in combination with medications depending on the severity and duration of symptoms. Pregnant individuals and healthcare providers collaborate to explore a range of treatment options and tailor care plans to meet individualized needs and preferences.

Education and Empowerment:

NPIs prioritize education, empowerment, and self-management skills for pregnant individuals, equipping them with knowledge, resources, and practical tools to navigate NVP symptoms with confidence and resilience. Pregnant individuals are encouraged to actively engage in self-care practices, seek support from healthcare providers, and advocate for their own well-being throughout the pregnancy journey.

Types of Non-Pharmaceutical Interventions (NPIs) Commonly Used for Managing Nausea and Vomiting in Pregnancy (NVP)

Non-pharmaceutical interventions (NPIs) offer pregnant individuals a variety of strategies and approaches to alleviate nausea and vomiting during pregnancy (NVP) without the use of traditional medications. In the book "Non-Pharmaceutical Interventions for Nausea and Vomiting in Pregnancy," several types of NPIs are commonly recommended and explored, each offering unique benefits and considerations. Here are some of the types of NPIs commonly used for managing NVP:

Dietary Modifications:

Dietary modifications involve adjusting food choices, meal timing, and portion sizes to help alleviate NVP symptoms. Recommendations may include consuming small, frequent meals rich in complex carbohydrates and lean proteins, avoiding spicy or greasy foods that may trigger nausea, and staying hydrated by sipping fluids throughout the day.

Hydration Strategies:

Hydration strategies focus on maintaining adequate fluid intake to prevent dehydration associated with vomiting and nausea. Pregnant individuals are encouraged to drink water, clear fluids, herbal teas, and electrolyte-rich beverages throughout the day, avoiding sugary or caffeinated drinks that may exacerbate symptoms.

Acupressure and Acupuncture:

Acupressure and acupuncture involve stimulating specific points on the body to alleviate nausea and vomiting. Techniques such as applying pressure to the P6 or Neiguan point on the inner wrist or receiving acupuncture treatments from a qualified practitioner may help reduce NVP symptoms and promote relaxation.

Ginger Supplementation:

Ginger supplementation is a natural remedy that has been studied for its anti-nausea properties. Pregnant individuals may consider incorporating ginger supplements, ginger tea, or ginger candies into their daily routine to help alleviate NVP symptoms. However, it is important to consult with a healthcare provider before using ginger supplements, especially at higher doses.

Aromatherapy: Aromatherapy involves using essential oils derived from plant extracts to promote relaxation and alleviate symptoms of nausea. Certain essential oils, such as peppermint, lemon, and lavender, may be diffused, diluted, or applied topically to help soothe NVP symptoms and enhance overall well-being.

Mindfulness and Relaxation Techniques: Mindfulness-based stress reduction techniques, relaxation exercises, and deep breathing techniques can help pregnant individuals manage stress, anxiety, and nausea associated with NVP. Practices such as yoga, meditation, guided imagery, and progressive muscle relaxation may promote a sense of calm and resilience during pregnancy.

Supportive Care and Peer Support: Emotional support from partners, family members, friends, and healthcare providers is invaluable for pregnant individuals experiencing NVP. Peer support groups, online forums, and community-based resources offer opportunities for pregnant individuals to connect with others facing similar challenges, share experiences, and access practical tips and coping strategies.

Evidence-Based Practices and Guidelines for Non-Pharmaceutical Interventions (NPIs)

In the book "Non-Pharmaceutical Interventions for Nausea and Vomiting in Pregnancy," the recommendations for NPIs are rooted in evidence-based practices and guidelines established by clinical research and expert consensus. These evidence-based practices serve as the foundation for developing comprehensive and effective strategies to manage nausea and vomiting during pregnancy (NVP). Here are some key evidence-based practices and guidelines for NPIs:

Dietary Modifications: Evidence suggests that dietary modifications can help alleviate NVP symptoms by minimizing triggers and promoting optimal nutrition. Recommendations typically include consuming small, frequent meals rich in complex carbohydrates and lean proteins, avoiding spicy or greasy foods that may exacerbate nausea, and staying hydrated by sipping fluids throughout the day.

Hydration Strategies:

Adequate hydration is essential for managing NVP and preventing dehydration associated with vomiting. Evidence-based hydration strategies include drinking water, clear fluids, herbal teas, and electrolyte-rich beverages throughout the day, avoiding sugary or caffeinated drinks that may worsen symptoms.

Acupressure and Acupuncture:

Research studies have shown that acupressure and acupuncture techniques, such as stimulating the P6 or Neiguan point on the inner wrist, can help reduce NVP symptoms and improve overall well-being. Evidence-based guidelines recommend incorporating these techniques into NVP management plans for pregnant individuals seeking non-pharmaceutical interventions.

Ginger Supplementation: Numerous clinical trials have investigated the efficacy of ginger supplementation in reducing NVP symptoms. Evidence suggests that ginger supplements, ginger tea, or ginger candies may help alleviate nausea and vomiting in pregnant individuals. However, it is important to consult with a healthcare provider before using ginger supplements, especially at higher doses.

Aromatherapy: While research on aromatherapy for NVP management is limited, certain essential oils, such as peppermint, lemon, and lavender, have been studied for their potential benefits. Evidence-based guidelines recommend cautious use of aromatherapy as a complementary approach to NPIs, emphasizing safety and individual preferences.

Mindfulness and Relaxation Techniques: Mindfulness-based stress reduction techniques, relaxation exercises, and deep breathing techniques have been shown to reduce stress and anxiety associated with NVP. Evidence-based guidelines advocate for incorporating these techniques into daily routines to promote emotional well-being and symptom relief during pregnancy.

Supportive Care and Peer Support:

Evidence suggests that emotional support from partners, family members, friends, and healthcare providers can have a positive impact on NVP management. Peer support groups, online forums, and community-based resources provide opportunities for pregnant individuals to share experiences, access practical tips, and seek encouragement from others facing similar challenges.

CHAPTER 3

DIETARY MODIFICATIONS AND NUTRITIONAL STRATEGIES

In the book "Non-Pharmaceutical Interventions for Nausea and Vomiting in Pregnancy," dietary modifications and nutritional strategies play a pivotal role in managing nausea and vomiting during pregnancy (NVP). By making informed choices about food intake and adopting nutritional strategies tailored to individual needs, pregnant individuals can alleviate symptoms, optimize nutrient intake, and improve overall well-being. Here are some key dietary modifications and nutritional strategies highlighted in the book:

Small, Frequent Meals: Consuming small, frequent meals throughout the day can help prevent gastric distension and alleviate NVP symptoms. Pregnant individuals are encouraged to eat every 2-3 hours, focusing on nutrient-dense foods that are easy to digest and tolerate.

Balanced Macronutrients:

Emphasizing a balance of macronutrients carbohydrates, proteins, and fats in each meal can help stabilize blood sugar levels and promote satiety. Complex carbohydrates such as whole grains, fruits, and vegetables, along with lean proteins and healthy fats, form the foundation of a nourishing diet during pregnancy.

Avoidance of Trigger Foods:

Identifying and avoiding trigger foods that exacerbate NVP symptoms is essential for managing discomfort and promoting gastrointestinal comfort. Spicy, fatty, or strongly flavored foods, as well as foods with strong odors, may trigger nausea and vomiting in susceptible individuals and should be minimized or avoided.

Hydration: Adequate hydration is crucial

for managing NVP and preventing dehydration associated with vomiting. Pregnant individuals are encouraged to sip fluids throughout the day, opting for water, herbal teas, electrolyte-rich beverages, and clear broths to replenish fluids and electrolytes lost through vomiting.

Nutrient-Rich Foods: Prioritizing nutrient-rich foods that provide essential vitamins, minerals, and antioxidants is important for supporting maternal and fetal health during pregnancy. Foods high in iron, calcium, vitamin D, vitamin B6, and folate, such as leafy greens, legumes, dairy products, lean meats, and fortified cereals, are integral components of a balanced diet.

Herbal Teas and Natural Remedies: Certain herbal teas and natural remedies may provide relief from NVP symptoms and promote gastrointestinal comfort. Ginger tea, peppermint tea, chamomile tea, and lemon balm tea are among the herbal remedies that pregnant individuals may find soothing and beneficial.

Nutritional Supplements: In cases where dietary intake is compromised due to severe NVP symptoms or food aversions, nutritional supplements may be recommended to bridge nutrient gaps and support maternal and fetal health. Prenatal vitamins containing folic acid, iron, calcium, vitamin D, and other essential nutrients are commonly prescribed to pregnant individuals as part of routine prenatal care.

Individualized Approach:

Recognizing that dietary preferences and tolerances vary among pregnant individuals, a personalized and individualized approach to dietary modifications and nutritional strategies is emphasized. Pregnant individuals are encouraged to work closely with healthcare providers, nutritionists, and dietitians to develop tailored meal plans that meet their unique needs and preferences.

The Importance of Diet in Managing Nausea and Vomiting in Pregnancy (NVP)

In the book "Non-Pharmaceutical Interventions for Nausea and Vomiting in Pregnancy," the significance of diet emerges as a cornerstone in the management of nausea and vomiting during pregnancy (NVP). Understanding the role of diet and implementing appropriate dietary modifications are essential components of non-pharmaceutical interventions aimed at alleviating NVP symptoms and promoting maternal well-being. Here are key points highlighting the importance of diet in managing NVP:

Nutritional Support:

Maintaining adequate nutrition is vital for supporting maternal health and fetal development during pregnancy. Despite experiencing NVP symptoms, pregnant individuals require essential nutrients to meet the increased demands of pregnancy. Dietary interventions focus on optimizing nutrient intake to mitigate the potential consequences of inadequate nutrition, such as maternal weight loss, nutritional deficiencies, and fetal growth restrictions.

Symptom Management:

Dietary modifications play a pivotal role in managing NVP symptoms by minimizing triggers and promoting gastric comfort. Certain foods and beverages may exacerbate nausea and vomiting, while others may provide relief and support digestive tolerance. Tailoring dietary choices to individual preferences and tolerances can help pregnant individuals identify foods that are well-tolerated and minimize discomfort during episodes of NVP.

Prevention of Gastric Distress:

NVP symptoms, including nausea and vomiting, can disrupt normal gastrointestinal function and contribute to gastric distress. Dietary strategies aim to prevent gastric distension and promote gastric comfort by advocating for small, frequent meals and snacks throughout the day. Consuming smaller portions helps mitigate feelings of fullness and reduces the likelihood of triggering NVP symptoms, allowing for better nutrient absorption and digestion.

Hydration and Fluid Balance:

Adequate hydration is crucial for managing NVP and preventing dehydration associated with vomiting and fluid losses. Pregnant individuals are encouraged to maintain hydration by sipping fluids regularly throughout the day, opting for clear liquids, electrolyte-rich beverages, and herbal teas. Hydration strategies complement dietary modifications and support overall well-being during pregnancy.

Optimization of Nutrient Absorption:

Selecting nutrient-dense foods and beverages enhances nutrient absorption and optimizes maternal-fetal health outcomes. Emphasizing whole foods rich in complex carbohydrates, lean proteins, healthy fats, vitamins, and minerals provides essential nutrients necessary for fetal development and maternal well-being. Incorporating a variety of nutrient sources promotes dietary diversity and ensures adequate nutrient intake despite NVP-related challenges.

Individualized Approach:

Recognizing the unique dietary preferences, aversions, and tolerances of pregnant individuals is integral to designing individualized dietary plans for managing NVP. Flexibility and adaptability are key principles in navigating dietary modifications, allowing pregnant individuals to explore alternative food options, experiment with meal timing and composition, and adjust dietary patterns based on evolving needs and experiences.

Dietary Modifications for Alleviating NVP Symptoms

Dietary modifications play a crucial role in managing nausea and vomiting in pregnancy (NVP). The relationship between nutrition and NVP is complex, with certain foods exacerbating symptoms while others provide relief. In this chapter, we explore specific dietary modifications that pregnant individuals can implement to alleviate NVP symptoms and promote overall well-being.

Importance of Diet in Managing NVP:

Dietary interventions offer pregnant individuals a non-pharmacological approach to managing NVP that is safe, accessible, and effective. The importance of diet in managing NVP lies in its potential to:

Minimize Triggers: Certain foods and dietary habits can trigger or exacerbate NVP symptoms. By identifying and avoiding these triggers, pregnant individuals can reduce the frequency and severity of nausea and vomiting episodes.

Provide Nutritional Support: Adequate nutrition is essential for maternal and fetal health during pregnancy. Despite experiencing NVP, pregnant individuals must maintain adequate nutrient intake to support fetal growth and development.

Improve Hydration: Dehydration can exacerbate NVP symptoms and increase the risk of complications such as electrolyte imbalances. Consuming hydrating foods and fluids can help maintain optimal hydration levels and prevent dehydration.

Enhance Overall Well-being: A balanced and nutritious diet can contribute to overall well-being by providing essential nutrients, stabilizing blood sugar levels, and promoting gastrointestinal health.

Specific Dietary Modifications to Alleviate Symptoms

Small, Frequent Meals: Consuming small, frequent meals throughout the day can help prevent stomach distension and minimize nausea and vomiting episodes.

57

Opt for light, easily digestible foods such as crackers, toast, fruits, and vegetables.

High-Protein Snacks: Protein-rich snacks, such as nuts, yogurt, cheese, and hard-boiled eggs, can help stabilize blood sugar levels and provide sustained energy throughout the day. Avoid high-fat and greasy snacks that may exacerbate NVP symptoms.

Complex Carbohydrates: Choose complex carbohydrates, such as whole grains, brown rice, quinoa, and oats, which provide sustained energy and promote satiety. Avoid refined carbohydrates and sugary foods that can cause blood sugar fluctuations and worsen nausea.

Ginger: Incorporate ginger into your diet through ginger tea, ginger candies, or ginger-infused recipes. Ginger has anti-nausea properties and may help alleviate NVP symptoms in some individuals.

Hydration: Stay hydrated by drinking water, herbal teas, coconut water, and electrolyte-rich beverages throughout the day. Sip fluids slowly to prevent discomfort and avoid large quantities of fluid during meals.

Avoid Trigger Foods: Identify and avoid foods that trigger or worsen NVP symptoms. Common triggers include spicy, greasy, and highly seasoned foods, as well as strong odors and flavors.

Consider Prenatal Supplements: In cases where dietary intake is compromised due to NVP, prenatal supplements prescribed by a healthcare provider can help bridge nutritional gaps and ensure adequate intake of essential vitamins and minerals.

Nutritional Supplements in NVP Management

Nutritional supplements play a vital role in managing nausea and vomiting in pregnancy (NVP) by addressing potential nutrient deficiencies and supporting maternal and fetal health. In this chapter, we explore the role of nutritional supplements in NVP management, including key nutrients, recommended supplements, and considerations for pregnant individuals.

59

Importance of Nutritional Supplements in NVP Management:

Addressing Nutrient Deficiencies: NVP can impact dietary intake and nutrient absorption, leading to potential deficiencies in essential vitamins and minerals critical for maternal and fetal health. Nutritional supplements help bridge these gaps and ensure optimal nutrient intake during pregnancy.

Supporting Fetal Development: Adequate nutrition is essential for fetal growth and development, particularly during the critical early stages of pregnancy. Nutritional supplements provide essential nutrients that support fetal organ development, neural tube formation, and overall growth.

Alleviating Symptoms: Certain vitamins and minerals have been shown to alleviate NVP symptoms and improve overall well-being. Nutritional supplements with anti-nausea properties, such as vitamin B6 and ginger, may help reduce nausea and vomiting episodes in pregnant individuals.

Preventing Complications: Nutritional deficiencies during pregnancy can increase the risk of complications such as preterm birth, low birth weight, and neural tube defects. Nutritional supplements help prevent these complications by ensuring adequate nutrient intake throughout pregnancy.

Recommended Nutritional Supplements for NVP Management:

Vitamin B6 (Pyridoxine): Vitamin B6 supplementation has been shown to reduce NVP symptoms, particularly when taken in combination with other nutrients. Pregnant individuals experiencing NVP may benefit from vitamin B6 supplements under the guidance of a healthcare provider.

Ginger: Ginger supplements or ginger-containing products, such as ginger tea or ginger candies, have been used for centuries to alleviate nausea and vomiting. Pregnant individuals may consider incorporating ginger supplements into their NVP management regimen, although dosing should be monitored and discussed with a healthcare provider.

61

Prenatal Vitamins: Prenatal vitamins are specially formulated multivitamin supplements designed to meet the unique nutritional needs of pregnant individuals. These supplements typically contain essential vitamins and minerals, including folic acid, iron, calcium, vitamin D, and omega-3 fatty acids, which are important for maternal and fetal health.

Considerations for Pregnant Individuals:

Consultation with Healthcare Provider: Pregnant individuals should consult with their healthcare provider before starting any nutritional supplements, including prenatal vitamins and herbal remedies. Healthcare providers can provide personalized recommendations based on individual nutritional needs and medical history.

Monitoring for Adverse Effects: While nutritional supplements are generally safe when taken as directed, pregnant individuals should be vigilant for any adverse effects or reactions. It is important to report any concerns or changes in symptoms to a healthcare provider promptly.

Balanced Diet: Nutritional supplements are intended to complement, not replace, a balanced diet rich in nutrient-dense foods. Pregnant individuals should focus on consuming a variety of fruits, vegetables, whole grains, lean proteins, and dairy products to support overall health and well-being.

CHAPTER 4

LIFESTYLE MODIFICATIONS AND BEHAVIORAL STRATEGIES FOR NVP MANAGEMENT

Lifestyle modifications and behavioral strategies are integral components of non-pharmaceutical interventions for managing nausea and vomiting in pregnancy (NVP). In this chapter, we delve into the various lifestyle changes and behavioral strategies that pregnant individuals can implement to alleviate NVP symptoms and improve their overall well-being.

Importance of Lifestyle Modifications and Behavioral Strategies in NVP Management:

Holistic Approach: Lifestyle modifications and behavioral strategies offer a holistic approach to NVP management by addressing the interconnected factors that contribute to nausea and vomiting during pregnancy. These interventions focus on enhancing overall health and well-being while minimizing discomfort associated with NVP.

Empowerment and Self-Care: By incorporating lifestyle modifications and behavioral strategies into their daily routines, pregnant individuals can take an active role in managing NVP symptoms and promoting their own well-being. These strategies empower individuals to make informed choices and adopt healthier habits during pregnancy.

Complementary to Medical Interventions: Lifestyle modifications and behavioral strategies complement medical interventions and may be used alone or in combination with pharmacological treatments depending on the severity and duration of NVP symptoms. These interventions provide additional tools for pregnant individuals to explore in their journey towards symptom relief.

Long-Term Health Benefits: Many lifestyle modifications and behavioral strategies promote long-term health benefits beyond alleviating NVP symptoms. By adopting healthy habits during pregnancy, individuals may reduce their risk of developing chronic conditions and promote positive health outcomes for themselves and their babies.

Recommended Lifestyle Modifications and Behavioral Strategies for NVP Management:

Stress Reduction Techniques: Stress and anxiety can exacerbate NVP symptoms. Pregnant individuals can benefit from stress reduction techniques such as mindfulness meditation, deep breathing exercises, progressive muscle relaxation, and guided imagery to promote relaxation and emotional well-being.

Adequate Rest and Sleep: Fatigue and inadequate sleep can contribute to increased nausea and vomiting during pregnancy. Pregnant individuals should prioritize adequate rest and sleep by establishing a consistent sleep schedule, practicing good sleep hygiene, and incorporating relaxation techniques before bedtime.

Regular Physical Activity: Moderate exercise, such as walking, swimming, yoga, and prenatal aerobics, can help alleviate NVP symptoms and improve overall physical and mental well-being. Pregnant individuals should consult with their healthcare provider to develop a safe and appropriate exercise routine tailored to their individual needs and abilities.

Avoiding Triggers: Identifying and avoiding triggers that exacerbate NVP symptoms can help pregnant individuals manage their condition more effectively. Common triggers include strong odors, spicy or greasy foods, fatigue, and dehydration. Pregnant individuals should take proactive steps to minimize exposure to these triggers whenever possible.

Nutritional Counseling: Working with a registered dietitian or nutritionist can help pregnant individuals develop personalized meal plans and dietary strategies to alleviate NVP symptoms while ensuring adequate nutrient intake for themselves and their babies. Nutrition counseling may include recommendations for small, frequent meals, hydration strategies, and dietary modifications to address individual needs and preferences.

Stress Reduction Techniques for NVP Management

Stress reduction techniques play a crucial role in managing nausea and vomiting in pregnancy (NVP) by addressing the emotional and physiological factors that contribute to symptom exacerbation. In this chapter, we explore various stress reduction techniques tailored to pregnant individuals experiencing NVP, offering practical strategies to promote relaxation, emotional well-being, and symptom relief.

Understanding the Impact of Stress on NVP:

Stress is known to exacerbate nausea and vomiting symptoms in pregnancy through its effects on the autonomic nervous system and gastrointestinal function. Pregnant individuals experiencing high levels of stress may be more susceptible to NVP episodes, leading to increased discomfort and reduced quality of life. By addressing stress through targeted interventions, pregnant individuals can mitigate its impact on NVP symptoms and overall well-being.

Stress Reduction Techniques:

Mindfulness Meditation: Mindfulness meditation involves focusing attention on the present moment without judgment, allowing pregnant individuals to cultivate awareness and acceptance of their thoughts, feelings, and bodily sensations. Mindfulness meditation practices, such as body scans, mindful breathing, and guided imagery, can help reduce stress, anxiety, and NVP symptoms.

Progressive Muscle Relaxation (PMR): Progressive muscle relaxation techniques involve systematically tensing and relaxing muscle groups throughout the body to promote physical and mental relaxation. Pregnant individuals can practice PMR exercises, starting from the toes and working their way up to the scalp, to release tension, alleviate stress, and promote overall well-being.

69

Deep Breathing Exercises: Deep breathing exercises, such as diaphragmatic breathing and belly breathing, focus on slow, rhythmic inhalation and exhalation to activate the body's relaxation response. Pregnant individuals can practice deep breathing techniques whenever they feel stressed, anxious, or overwhelmed, using the breath as a tool to calm the mind and body.

Yoga and Gentle Stretching: Yoga and gentle stretching routines tailored to pregnancy offer pregnant individuals an opportunity to connect with their bodies, release tension, and cultivate relaxation. Prenatal yoga classes and online resources provide safe and effective practices that support physical and emotional well-being during pregnancy.

Creative Expression: Engaging in creative activities, such as journaling, drawing, painting, or listening to music, can provide pregnant individuals with an outlet for self-expression and emotional processing. Creative expression allows individuals to explore their thoughts and emotions, fostering a sense of empowerment and resilience in the face of NVP challenges.

Social Support and Connection: Seeking support from partners, family members, friends, and healthcare providers can help pregnant individuals navigate the emotional ups and downs of NVP. Sharing experiences, seeking reassurance, and expressing feelings of vulnerability can strengthen social connections and promote emotional well-being during pregnancy.

Relaxation Exercises and Mindfulness Practices

Managing nausea and vomiting in pregnancy (NVP) involves not only physical interventions but also strategies to promote mental and emotional well-being. In this chapter, we delve into relaxation exercises and mindfulness practices as non-pharmaceutical interventions for alleviating NVP symptoms and enhancing overall pregnancy experience.

71

Importance of Relaxation Exercises and Mindfulness Practices:

Pregnancy can be a time of heightened stress and anxiety, particularly for individuals experiencing NVP symptoms. Relaxation exercises and mindfulness practices offer pregnant individuals valuable tools to manage stress, reduce anxiety, and cultivate a sense of calm amidst the challenges of NVP.

Relaxation Exercises:

Deep Breathing Techniques: Deep breathing exercises involve slow, deliberate inhalation and exhalation to promote relaxation and reduce stress. Pregnant individuals can practice deep breathing techniques in various positions, such as seated, lying down, or during prenatal yoga sessions.

Progressive Muscle Relaxation (PMR): PMR involves tensing and relaxing different muscle groups in the body to release tension and promote physical relaxation. Pregnant individuals can systematically tense and relax muscles from head to toe, focusing on areas of tension and discomfort.

Guided Imagery: Guided imagery exercises involve visualizing peaceful and calming scenes to evoke feelings of relaxation and well-being. Pregnant individuals can listen to guided imagery recordings or create their own mental imagery to transport themselves to serene and tranquil environments.

Mindfulness Practices:

Meditation: Meditation involves focusing attention on the present moment without judgment, allowing thoughts and sensations to arise and pass without attachment. Pregnant individuals can practice mindfulness meditation through guided meditations, breath awareness exercises, or silent meditation sessions.

Body Scan Meditation: Body scan meditation involves systematically bringing awareness to different parts of the body, observing sensations, and cultivating a sense of acceptance and presence. Pregnant individuals can practice body scan meditation to connect with their bodies and promote relaxation.

Mindful Movement:

Mindful movement practices, such as prenatal yoga, tai chi, or gentle stretching exercises, combine physical activity with mindfulness techniques to promote relaxation and stress reduction. Pregnant individuals can engage in mindful movement practices tailored to their comfort level and physical abilities.

Integration into Daily Routine:

Incorporating relaxation exercises and mindfulness practices into daily routine can enhance their effectiveness in managing NVP symptoms and promoting overall well-being. Pregnant individuals are encouraged to set aside dedicated time each day for relaxation and mindfulness practices, whether it be in the morning, during breaks throughout the day, or before bedtime.

Relaxation Exercises and Mindfulness Practices for Nausea and Vomiting in Pregnancy

Relaxation exercises and mindfulness practices offer valuable tools for managing nausea and vomiting in pregnancy (NVP) by promoting emotional well-being, reducing stress, and enhancing coping skills. In this chapter, we explore various relaxation techniques and mindfulness practices that pregnant individuals can incorporate into their daily routines to alleviate NVP symptoms and improve overall quality of life.

Relaxation Exercises:

Deep Breathing Techniques: Deep breathing exercises involve slow, deliberate inhalation and exhalation to promote relaxation and reduce stress. Pregnant individuals can practice deep breathing by inhaling deeply through the nose, holding the breath for a few seconds, and exhaling slowly through the mouth. Repeat this process several times to induce a state of calmness and relaxation.

Progressive Muscle Relaxation (PMR): PMR is a relaxation technique that involves systematically tensing and relaxing different muscle groups in the body. Pregnant individuals can start by tensing the muscles in their feet and gradually working their way up to the muscles in their legs, abdomen, arms, and face. By systematically releasing tension throughout the body, PMR helps reduce physical discomfort and promote relaxation.

Guided Imagery: Guided imagery involves visualizing calming and peaceful scenes to promote relaxation and reduce stress. Pregnant individuals can close their eyes and imagine themselves in a serene natural setting, such as a tranquil beach or a lush forest. By focusing on positive imagery and engaging the senses, guided imagery can help distract from NVP symptoms and induce a sense of relaxation.

Mindfulness Practices:

Mindful Breathing: Mindful breathing involves focusing attention on the sensations of breathing, such as the rise and fall of the chest and the feeling of air passing through the nostrils. Pregnant individuals can practice mindful breathing by observing each breath without judgment or attachment to thoughts or emotions. Mindful breathing helps cultivate present-moment awareness and reduces reactivity to NVP symptoms.

Body Scan Meditation: Body scan meditation is a mindfulness practice that involves systematically directing attention to different parts of the body, from the toes to the crown of the head. Pregnant individuals can practice body scan meditation by bringing awareness to sensations, tensions, and areas of discomfort in the body. By cultivating non-judgmental awareness and acceptance of bodily sensations, body scan meditation promotes relaxation and reduces stress.

Mindful Eating: Mindful eating involves paying attention to the sensory experiences and physical sensations associated with eating, such as taste, texture, and fullness. Pregnant individuals can practice mindful eating by savoring each bite, chewing slowly, and noticing the flavors and aromas of food. By fostering a

77

mindful relationship with food, mindful eating can help reduce nausea, improve digestion, and enhance overall well-being.

CHAPTER 5

SLEEP HYGIENE AND ITS IMPACT ON NAUSEA AND VOMITING IN PREGNANCY (NVP)

Sleep hygiene refers to a set of practices and habits that promote healthy sleep patterns and improve the quality of sleep. Adequate sleep hygiene is essential for overall well-being, particularly during pregnancy when sleep disturbances are common. In this chapter, we explore the importance of sleep hygiene and its impact on nausea and vomiting in pregnancy (NVP).

The Importance of Sleep Hygiene in NVP Management:

Hormonal Changes: During pregnancy, hormonal fluctuations, particularly changes in progesterone levels, can disrupt sleep patterns and contribute to feelings of fatigue and nausea. Maintaining good sleep hygiene can help mitigate the impact of hormonal changes on NVP symptoms.

Stress Reduction: **Poor sleep quality and inadequate sleep duration can increase stress levels and exacerbate NVP symptoms. By prioritizing sleep hygiene practices, pregnant individuals can reduce stress, promote relaxation, and improve their ability to cope with NVP-related discomfort.**

Immune Function: **Adequate sleep is essential for maintaining a healthy immune system and reducing inflammation in the body. Poor sleep hygiene may compromise immune function, making pregnant individuals more susceptible to infections and illnesses that can exacerbate NVP symptoms.**

Energy Levels: **Quality sleep is essential for restoring energy levels and promoting physical and mental well-being. Pregnant individuals who prioritize sleep hygiene are more likely to experience increased energy levels and improved overall functioning, which can help alleviate NVP-related fatigue and lethargy.**

Impact of Sleep Hygiene Practices on NVP:

Establishing a Consistent Sleep Schedule: Going to bed and waking up at the same time each day helps regulate the body's internal clock and promotes healthy sleep-wake cycles. Pregnant individuals are encouraged to establish a consistent sleep schedule to optimize sleep quality and reduce NVP symptoms.

Creating a Restful Sleep Environment:

A conducive sleep environment is essential for promoting relaxation and improving sleep quality. Pregnant individuals should create a cool, dark, and quiet sleep environment free from distractions, such as electronic devices and excessive noise, to enhance restfulness and alleviate NVP-related discomfort.

Practicing Relaxation Techniques:

Relaxation techniques, such as deep breathing, progressive muscle relaxation, and guided imagery, can help pregnant individuals unwind before bedtime and promote restful sleep.

Integrating relaxation practices into bedtime routines can reduce stress, anxiety, and NVP symptoms, improving overall sleep quality.

Addressing Discomfort: Pregnancy-related discomfort, such as back pain, heartburn, and frequent urination, can disrupt sleep and exacerbate NVP symptoms. Pregnant individuals are encouraged to use supportive pillows, adjust sleeping positions, and address any underlying discomfort to improve sleep quality and alleviate NVP-related issues.

Alternative Therapies and Complementary Medicine for Nausea and Vomiting in Pregnancy

Alternative therapies and complementary medicine offer pregnant individuals non-pharmacological approaches to managing nausea and vomiting in pregnancy (NVP). In this chapter, we explore various alternative therapies and complementary medicine modalities that may alleviate NVP symptoms and promote overall well-being.

Acupuncture: Acupuncture involves the insertion of thin needles into specific points on the body to restore balance and promote healing. Research suggests that acupuncture may help alleviate NVP symptoms by regulating hormonal imbalances and reducing nausea and vomiting episodes. Pregnant individuals considering acupuncture should seek treatment from a qualified and experienced acupuncturist who specializes in prenatal care.

Acupressure: Acupressure is a non-invasive alternative therapy that involves applying pressure to specific acupoints on the body to relieve symptoms and promote wellness. The P6 or Neiguan point, located on the inner wrist, is commonly targeted for NVP management. Pregnant individuals can use acupressure wristbands or apply gentle pressure to the P6 point to help alleviate nausea and vomiting episodes.

Herbal Remedies: Certain herbal remedies, such as ginger and peppermint, have been traditionally used to alleviate nausea and promote digestive health. Ginger supplements, ginger tea, and peppermint oil may help reduce NVP symptoms in some pregnant individuals. However, it is essential to consult with a healthcare provider before using herbal remedies during pregnancy to ensure safety and efficacy.

Aromatherapy: Aromatherapy involves the use of essential oils derived from plants to promote relaxation, reduce stress, and alleviate symptoms. Essential oils such as peppermint, lemon, and lavender may help alleviate NVP symptoms when used in diffusers, massage oils, or inhalers. Pregnant individuals should exercise caution when using essential oils and consult with a qualified aromatherapist or healthcare provider.

Homeopathy: Homeopathy is a holistic system of medicine based on the principle of "like cures like," where highly diluted substances are used to stimulate the body's innate healing response. Homeopathic remedies such as Nux vomica and Ipecacuanha may be recommended for NVP management based on individual symptoms and constitutional factors. Pregnant individuals should consult with a qualified homeopath to determine the most appropriate remedies for their needs.

Acupressure and Acupuncture: Alternative Therapies for Nausea and Vomiting in Pregnancy

Acupressure and acupuncture are alternative therapies rooted in traditional Chinese medicine that have gained recognition for their potential effectiveness in managing nausea and vomiting in pregnancy (NVP). In this chapter, we explore the principles, techniques, and evidence supporting the use of acupressure and acupuncture as non-pharmaceutical interventions for NVP.

Principles of Acupressure and Acupuncture:

Traditional Chinese Medicine (TCM) Principles: Acupressure and acupuncture are based on the principles of Traditional Chinese Medicine, which views the body as interconnected energy channels, or meridians, through which vital energy, or Qi, flows. Imbalances or blockages in Qi flow are believed to contribute to health conditions, including NVP.

Acupressure: Acupressure involves applying pressure to specific acupoints along the body's meridians using fingers, thumbs, or specialized devices. By stimulating acupoints associated with nausea and vomiting, acupressure aims to restore balance and alleviate symptoms.

Acupuncture: Acupuncture involves inserting thin needles into specific acupoints to stimulate Qi flow and rebalance the body's energy. Acupuncture points selected for NVP management target areas associated with gastrointestinal function, stress reduction, and hormonal regulation.

Evidence Supporting Acupressure and Acupuncture for NVP:

Clinical Studies: Numerous clinical studies have investigated the effectiveness of acupressure and acupuncture for NVP management, with many reporting positive outcomes, including reduced nausea and vomiting frequency and severity.

Meta-Analyses: Meta-analyses of randomized controlled trials have provided further support for the efficacy of acupressure and acupuncture in alleviating NVP symptoms. These analyses have demonstrated statistically significant reductions in nausea and vomiting scores among pregnant individuals receiving acupressure or acupuncture compared to control groups.

Mechanisms of Action: The mechanisms underlying the effectiveness of acupressure and acupuncture for NVP management are not fully understood but may involve modulation of neurotransmitter levels, regulation of hormonal pathways, and stimulation of the body's natural healing mechanisms.

Practical Considerations for Acupressure and Acupuncture in Pregnancy:

Safety: Acupressure and acupuncture are generally considered safe when performed by trained practitioners using sterile needles and appropriate techniques. Pregnant individuals should seek qualified acupressure or acupuncture practitioners experienced in working with pregnant clients.

Individualized Treatment: Acupressure and acupuncture treatments should be tailored to the unique needs and preferences of pregnant individuals. Treatment frequency, duration, and acupoint selection may vary based on symptom severity, gestational age, and individual response.

Consultation with Healthcare Provider: Pregnant individuals considering acupressure or acupuncture for NVP management should consult with their healthcare provider to discuss potential benefits, risks, and contraindications. Healthcare providers can offer guidance and support to ensure safe and effective integration of alternative therapies into comprehensive care plans.

Herbal Remedies and Aromatherapy for Managing Nausea and Vomiting in Pregnancy

Herbal remedies and aromatherapy offer alternative approaches to managing nausea and vomiting in pregnancy (NVP) without the use of traditional medications. In this chapter, we explore the potential benefits, safety considerations, and practical applications of herbal remedies and aromatherapy for pregnant individuals experiencing NVP.

Herbal Remedies:

Ginger (Zingiber officinale): Ginger is one of the most widely studied herbal remedies for NVP and is known for its anti-nausea properties. Pregnant individuals may benefit from consuming ginger in various forms, including fresh ginger root, ginger tea, ginger candies, and ginger supplements. However, it is important to consult with a healthcare provider before using ginger supplements, especially at higher doses.

Peppermint (Mentha piperita): Peppermint is another herb commonly used to alleviate nausea and digestive discomfort. Pregnant individuals can enjoy peppermint tea or inhale peppermint essential oil to help relieve NVP symptoms. However, peppermint oil should be used with caution, as high doses may cause heartburn or exacerbate acid reflux.

Lemon Balm (Melissa officinalis): Lemon balm is a calming herb that may help reduce anxiety and relieve nausea. Pregnant individuals can brew lemon balm tea or use lemon balm essential oil in aromatherapy to promote relaxation and alleviate NVP-related discomfort.

Aromatherapy:

Peppermint Essential Oil: Peppermint essential oil is known for its invigorating scent and digestive benefits. Pregnant individuals can diffuse peppermint oil in their living spaces or inhale it directly from the bottle to help alleviate NVP symptoms. Peppermint oil should be used in moderation, as excessive inhalation may cause adverse reactions.

Lemon Essential Oil: Lemon essential oil has a refreshing aroma and may help reduce feelings of nausea and vomiting. Pregnant individuals can add a few drops of lemon oil to a diffuser or inhale it from the bottle to promote relaxation and alleviate NVP-related discomfort.

Lavender Essential Oil: Lavender essential oil is prized for its calming and soothing properties. Pregnant individuals can use lavender oil in aromatherapy by diffusing it in their bedrooms or adding a few drops to a warm bath. Lavender oil may help reduce stress, anxiety, and NVP symptoms.

Safety Considerations:

Consultation with Healthcare Provider: Pregnant individuals should consult with their healthcare providers before using herbal remedies or aromatherapy for NVP management. While many herbs and essential oils are considered safe during pregnancy, some may pose risks or interact with medications.

Quality and Purity: It is important to choose high-quality herbal products and essential oils from reputable sources to ensure purity and potency. Pregnant individuals should avoid products containing additives, fillers, or synthetic ingredients that may compromise safety.

Individual Sensitivities: Pregnant individuals may have individual sensitivities or allergies to certain herbs or essential oils. It is essential to perform a patch test and monitor for any adverse reactions when using herbal remedies or aromatherapy for NVP management.

Yoga and Mind-Body Interventions for Managing Nausea and Vomiting in Pregnancy

Yoga and other mind-body interventions offer holistic approaches to managing nausea and vomiting in pregnancy (NVP) by integrating physical postures, breathing techniques, relaxation exercises, and mindfulness practices. In this chapter, we explore the potential benefits, safety considerations, and practical applications of yoga and mind-body interventions for pregnant individuals experiencing NVP.

Yoga:

Gentle Yoga Poses: Gentle yoga poses, such as cat-cow stretch, child's pose, and seated twists, can help alleviate tension, improve circulation, and promote relaxation in pregnant individuals experiencing NVP. Modified yoga poses tailored to accommodate the changing needs of pregnancy can provide gentle stretches and release tension in the body.

Breathing Techniques: Pranayama, or yogic breathing techniques, can help pregnant individuals manage stress, reduce anxiety, and alleviate NVP symptoms. Deep breathing exercises, such as abdominal breathing and alternate nostril breathing, promote relaxation, increase oxygenation, and enhance overall well-being during pregnancy.

Meditation and Mindfulness: Meditation and mindfulness practices cultivate present-moment awareness, reduce reactivity to NVP symptoms, and promote emotional well-being in pregnant individuals. Mindful meditation techniques, such as body scan meditation, loving-kindness meditation, and guided imagery, help pregnant individuals develop resilience and cope with NVP-related discomfort.

Other Mind-Body Interventions:

Progressive Muscle Relaxation (PMR): PMR involves systematically tensing and relaxing different muscle groups in the body to reduce tension, promote relaxation, and alleviate NVP symptoms. Pregnant individuals can practice PMR by sequentially tensing and releasing muscles from the feet to the head, focusing on each sensation and letting go of muscular tension.

Guided Imagery and Visualization: Guided imagery and visualization techniques involve mentally conjuring calming and peaceful scenes to reduce stress, alleviate nausea, and promote relaxation in pregnant individuals. Guided imagery scripts and visualization exercises tailored to pregnancy-related themes can help pregnant individuals create positive mental images and cope with NVP-related discomfort.

Safety Considerations:

Consultation with Healthcare Provider: Pregnant individuals should consult with their healthcare providers before starting any new exercise or mind-body intervention program, including yoga and meditation. Healthcare providers can offer guidance, address concerns, and ensure that mind-body interventions are safe and appropriate for the individual's pregnancy.

Modification and Adaptation: Pregnant individuals should modify yoga poses and mind-body practices to accommodate the changing needs and limitations of pregnancy. Avoiding strenuous or high-impact activities, practicing gentle movements, and listening to the body's signals are essential for ensuring safety and minimizing discomfort during mind-body interventions.

Hydration and Rest: Pregnant individuals participating in yoga and mind-body interventions should stay hydrated, take breaks as needed, and prioritize rest and relaxation. Overexertion and dehydration can exacerbate NVP symptoms and compromise maternal and fetal well-being during pregnancy.

CHAPTER 6

SUPPORTIVE CARE AND PRACTICAL TIPS FOR MANAGING NAUSEA AND VOMITING IN PREGNANCY

Supportive care and practical tips are essential components of managing nausea and vomiting in pregnancy (NVP), providing pregnant individuals with guidance, resources, and emotional support to cope with NVP-related challenges. In this chapter, we explore various supportive care strategies and practical tips for pregnant individuals experiencing NVP.

Supportive Care Strategies:

Emotional Support: Pregnant individuals experiencing NVP benefit from emotional support from partners, family members, friends, and healthcare providers. Creating a supportive and understanding environment where pregnant individuals feel comfortable expressing their concerns, fears, and frustrations can help alleviate emotional distress and promote well-being.

Peer Support Groups: Peer support groups and online forums provide pregnant individuals with opportunities to connect with others facing similar challenges, share experiences, and exchange practical tips for managing NVP. Peer support fosters a sense of community, validation, and empowerment, reducing feelings of isolation and promoting resilience.

Healthcare Provider Collaboration: Collaborating with healthcare providers, including obstetricians, midwives, and registered dietitians, is essential for developing personalized NVP management plans tailored to the individual's needs and preferences. Healthcare providers offer guidance, monitor maternal and fetal well-being, and provide evidence-based interventions to alleviate NVP symptoms and promote overall health.

Practical Tips for Managing NVP:

Dietary Modifications: Implementing dietary modifications, such as consuming small, frequent meals, avoiding trigger foods, and staying hydrated, can help alleviate NVP symptoms and maintain adequate nutrition during pregnancy. Pregnant individuals should experiment with different food choices and eating patterns to identify strategies that minimize discomfort and promote well-being.

Rest and Relaxation: Prioritizing rest and relaxation is essential for managing NVP-related fatigue, stress, and discomfort. Pregnant individuals should listen to their bodies, take breaks as needed, and engage in activities that promote relaxation, such as meditation, gentle exercise, and leisure activities.

Acupressure Bands: Acupressure bands, such as Sea-Bands, apply pressure to the P6 or Neiguan point on the inner wrist, potentially reducing NVP symptoms. Pregnant individuals can wear acupressure bands throughout the day or during times of increased nausea and vomiting to help alleviate discomfort.

Environmental Modifications: Making environmental modifications, such as

99

avoiding strong odors, minimizing exposure to triggers, and ensuring adequate ventilation, can help reduce NVP symptoms and improve overall comfort. Pregnant individuals should create a supportive and nurturing environment that promotes relaxation and well-being.

Emotional Support for Pregnant Individuals Experiencing Nausea and Vomiting in Pregnancy (NVP)

Emotional support plays a crucial role in helping pregnant individuals cope with the challenges of nausea and vomiting in pregnancy (NVP). In this chapter, we explore the importance of emotional support, strategies for providing support, and practical tips for managing NVP-related distress.

Understanding the Emotional Impact of NVP:

Anxiety and Stress: NVP can cause significant anxiety and stress for pregnant individuals, impacting their emotional well-being and quality of life. Fear of nausea episodes, uncertainty about symptom severity, and concerns about the impact on daily activities can contribute to emotional distress.

Feelings of Isolation: Pregnant individuals experiencing NVP may feel isolated and alone in their struggles, especially if they perceive that others do not understand or validate their experiences. Social withdrawal and reluctance to seek support can further exacerbate feelings of isolation and distress.

Impact on Mental Health: Persistent NVP symptoms can take a toll on mental health, leading to feelings of frustration, helplessness, and depression. Pregnant individuals may experience mood swings, irritability, and difficulty coping with everyday stressors as a result of NVP-related emotional strain.

Strategies for Providing Emotional Support:

Active Listening: Empathetic and non-judgmental listening is essential for providing effective emotional support to pregnant individuals experiencing NVP. Encourage open communication, validate their experiences, and acknowledge the challenges they are facing without minimizing their concerns.

Validation and Empathy: Validate the feelings and experiences of pregnant individuals experiencing NVP by acknowledging the impact of their symptoms on their daily lives and emotional well-being. Offer empathy and reassurance that their experiences are valid and worthy of support and understanding.

Practical Assistance: Offer practical assistance and support to pregnant individuals struggling with NVP, such as helping with household chores, running errands, or providing childcare support. Simple gestures of kindness and practical assistance can alleviate stress and lighten the burden of NVP-related challenges.

Practical Tips for Managing NVP-Related Distress:

Self-Care Practices: Encourage pregnant individuals to prioritize self-care practices that promote emotional well-being, such as engaging in relaxation techniques, practicing mindfulness, and taking breaks to rest and recharge.

Peer Support Networks: Connect pregnant individuals with peer support networks, online forums, or support groups where they can connect with others facing similar challenges, share experiences, and access practical tips and coping strategies for managing NVP.

Open Communication: Foster open and honest communication between pregnant individuals and their healthcare providers to discuss concerns, explore treatment options, and develop personalized strategies for managing NVP symptoms and emotional distress.

Practical Tips for Managing Nausea and Vomiting in Pregnancy (NVP) at Home and Work

Managing nausea and vomiting in pregnancy (NVP) can be challenging, especially when navigating daily responsibilities at home and work. In this chapter, we explore practical tips and strategies to help pregnant individuals effectively cope with NVP symptoms in both home and work environments.

Practical Tips for Managing NVP Symptoms at Home:

Dietary Modifications:

Eat small, frequent meals throughout the day to prevent stomach distension and reduce nausea.

Choose bland, easily digestible foods such as crackers, toast, and rice to minimize NVP symptoms.

Keep snacks such as crackers, ginger candies, and nuts readily available for quick relief.

Hydration:

Stay hydrated by sipping fluids like water, herbal teas, and electrolyte-rich drinks throughout the day.

Avoid drinking large amounts of fluids during meals, as it may exacerbate nausea and vomiting.

Rest and Relaxation:

Prioritize rest and relaxation by taking short naps or breaks during the day to alleviate fatigue and stress.

Practice relaxation techniques such as deep breathing, guided imagery, or meditation to promote a sense of calmness and well-being.

Support System:

Seek support from family members, friends, and partners who can offer practical assistance and emotional support during challenging times.

Communicate openly with loved ones about your NVP symptoms and how they can best support you at home.

Practical Tips for Managing NVP Symptoms at Work:

Flexible Work Arrangements:

Explore flexible work arrangements such as telecommuting, flexible hours, or modified duties with your employer to accommodate NVP-related challenges.

Communicate with your supervisor or human resources department about your

NVP symptoms and any necessary accommodations.

Nausea Relief Strategies:

Keep nausea relief essentials such as ginger candies, peppermint tea bags, and crackers at your workplace for quick access.

Take short breaks as needed to rest, hydrate, and alleviate nausea symptoms throughout the workday.

Minimize Triggers:

Identify and minimize triggers in your work environment that may exacerbate NVP symptoms, such as strong odors, fluorescent lighting, or prolonged screen time.

Create a comfortable and supportive workspace by adjusting lighting, temperature, and seating arrangements to reduce discomfort.

Supportive Colleagues:

Inform trusted colleagues or supervisors about your NVP symptoms and any accommodations you may require at work.

Seek understanding and support from colleagues who can offer assistance or cover for you during periods of increased NVP symptoms.

Importance of Communication with Healthcare Providers

Effective communication between pregnant individuals and their healthcare providers is paramount in the management of nausea and vomiting in pregnancy (NVP). In this chapter, we explore the importance of open, honest, and proactive communication in addressing NVP symptoms, ensuring maternal and fetal well-being, and promoting positive pregnancy experiences.

The Importance of Communication with Healthcare Providers:

Individualized Care: Each pregnancy is unique, and the severity and impact of NVP symptoms can vary significantly among pregnant individuals. Open communication with healthcare providers allows for the customization of care plans tailored to the specific needs, preferences, and circumstances of each individual.

Assessment and Monitoring: Regular communication with healthcare providers enables the ongoing assessment and monitoring of NVP symptoms, maternal health, and fetal well-being throughout pregnancy. Healthcare providers can evaluate the severity of symptoms, identify potential complications, and adjust management strategies accordingly.

Treatment Options: Healthcare providers can provide valuable insights into the available treatment options for managing NVP symptoms, including non-pharmaceutical interventions, dietary modifications, lifestyle changes, and, when necessary, pharmacological therapies. Open dialogue allows pregnant individuals to make informed decisions about their care and treatment preferences.

Emotional Support: NVP can have a significant impact on emotional well-being, quality of life, and maternal mental health. Healthcare providers play a vital role in offering emotional support, validation, and reassurance to pregnant individuals experiencing NVP-related distress, anxiety, or depression.

Practical Tips for Effective Communication:

Be Honest and Transparent: Share your NVP symptoms, concerns, and experiences openly and honestly with your healthcare provider. Providing accurate information allows healthcare providers to assess your condition comprehensively and develop appropriate management strategies.

Ask Questions: Do not hesitate to ask questions or seek clarification about NVP management, treatment options, potential side effects, and expectations. Understanding your care plan and treatment options empowers you to actively participate in your healthcare decisions.

Keep a Symptom Journal: Keeping a journal or diary of your NVP symptoms, triggers, and responses to interventions can provide valuable insights for healthcare providers. Documenting your experiences helps track symptom patterns, identify potential triggers, and monitor changes in symptom severity over time.

Discuss Concerns and Preferences: Share any concerns, preferences, or goals related to NVP management with your healthcare provider. Discuss your preferences for non-pharmaceutical interventions, dietary modifications, and lifestyle changes, and collaborate with your healthcare provider to develop a personalized care plan that aligns with your needs and preferences.

CHAPTER 7

EVALUATING EFFECTIVENESS AND SAFETY OF NON-PHARMACEUTICAL INTERVENTIONS (NPIS)

Assessing the effectiveness and safety of non-pharmaceutical interventions (NPIs) is crucial for optimizing the management of nausea and vomiting in pregnancy (NVP) while ensuring the well-being of both the pregnant individual and the fetus. In this chapter, we delve into the methodologies and considerations involved in evaluating the efficacy and safety of NPIs for NVP.

Clinical Trials and Studies:

Randomized controlled trials (RCTs) are considered the gold standard for evaluating the efficacy and safety of NPIs for NVP. RCTs involve randomly assigning participants to receive either the intervention or a control treatment, allowing for the comparison of outcomes between groups.

Prospective cohort studies and observational studies can also provide valuable insights into the effectiveness and safety of NPIs by following participants over time and monitoring outcomes associated with the interventions.

Outcome Measures:

Primary outcome measures in NVP studies often include the frequency and severity of nausea and vomiting episodes, as well as measures of maternal quality of life, functional status, and psychological well-being.

Secondary outcome measures may encompass factors such as dietary intake, hydration status, maternal weight gain, fetal outcomes, and adverse events related to the intervention.

Safety Monitoring:

Safety considerations are paramount in evaluating NPIs for NVP, particularly during pregnancy when the well-being of the fetus must be carefully safeguarded.

Adverse events, including maternal and fetal complications, side effects, and tolerability of interventions, should be systematically monitored and documented throughout the duration of the study.

Patient-reported Outcomes:

Patient-reported outcomes (PROs) offer insights into the subjective experiences and perceptions of pregnant individuals receiving NPIs for NVP.

Surveys, questionnaires, and structured interviews can be used to assess PROs related to symptom relief, treatment satisfaction, perceived effectiveness, and overall treatment experience.

Long-term Follow-up:

Long-term follow-up studies are essential for assessing the sustained effectiveness and safety of NPIs beyond the duration of the initial intervention.

Longitudinal studies that track outcomes over an extended period can identify any potential late-emerging effects, relapse of symptoms, or changes in treatment response over time.

Methods for Assessing the Effectiveness of Non-Pharmaceutical Interventions (NPIs) in Managing Nausea and Vomiting in Pregnancy (NVP)

Assessing the effectiveness of non-pharmaceutical interventions (NPIs) in managing nausea and vomiting in pregnancy (NVP) is critical for providing evidence-based care and optimizing treatment outcomes for pregnant individuals. In this chapter, we explore various methods and strategies for evaluating the effectiveness of NPIs in NVP management.

Randomized Controlled Trials (RCTs):

RCTs are considered the gold standard for assessing the effectiveness of NPIs in NVP management. Participants are randomly assigned to receive either the intervention or a control treatment (placebo or standard care), minimizing bias and allowing for the comparison of outcomes between groups.

RCTs typically involve predefined outcome measures, such as the frequency and severity of nausea and vomiting episodes, maternal quality of life, and adverse events associated with the intervention.

Prospective Cohort Studies:

Prospective cohort studies follow a group of pregnant individuals over time, collecting data on exposure to NPIs and outcomes related to NVP management.

Cohort studies allow researchers to assess the real-world effectiveness of NPIs in diverse populations and settings, providing valuable insights into treatment outcomes and long-term effects.

Case-Control Studies:

Case-control studies compare pregnant individuals with NVP who received a specific NPI (cases) to those who did not receive the intervention (controls), analyzing differences in outcomes between groups.

Case-control studies are particularly useful for investigating rare or severe outcomes associated with NVP management and identifying potential risk factors or protective factors.

Systematic Reviews and Meta-Analyses:

Systematic reviews and meta-analyses compile and analyze data from multiple studies to provide a comprehensive overview of the effectiveness of NPIs in NVP management.

By synthesizing evidence from various studies, systematic reviews and meta-analyses can offer insights into treatment efficacy, safety, and consistency across different populations and interventions.

Patient-Reported Outcome Measures (PROMs):

PROMs capture the subjective experiences and perspectives of pregnant individuals receiving NPIs for NVP, including symptom relief, treatment satisfaction, and quality of life.

Surveys, questionnaires, and standardized instruments are used to assess PROMs, allowing researchers to incorporate patient perspectives into effectiveness evaluations.

Longitudinal Studies:

Longitudinal studies track pregnant individuals over an extended period, assessing the sustained effectiveness and durability of NPIs in NVP management.

Longitudinal data collection allows researchers to evaluate treatment response over time, identify patterns of symptom recurrence or remission, and explore factors influencing treatment outcomes.

Safety Considerations and Potential Risks of Non-Pharmaceutical Interventions (NPIs)

While non-pharmaceutical interventions (NPIs) offer promising avenues for managing nausea and vomiting in pregnancy (NVP), it's crucial to carefully evaluate their safety profiles and potential risks. In this chapter, we examine safety considerations associated with various NPIs used in the management of NVP, providing insights into mitigating risks and optimizing maternal and fetal well-being.

117

Herbal Remedies:

Safety concerns exist regarding the use of certain herbal remedies for NVP, as their efficacy and safety profiles are not well-established through rigorous scientific research.

Some herbal remedies, such as ginger and peppermint, are generally considered safe when used in moderate amounts. However, high doses or prolonged use may pose risks, including gastrointestinal upset, allergic reactions, and potential interactions with medications.

Pregnant individuals should exercise caution and consult with healthcare providers before using herbal remedies to ensure safety and minimize potential risks to themselves and their babies.

Aromatherapy:

Aromatherapy involves the use of essential oils derived from plants to promote relaxation and alleviate symptoms. While generally considered safe when used appropriately, essential oils can be potent and may cause adverse reactions if misused.

Pregnant individuals should be cautious when using aromatherapy during pregnancy, as some essential oils may trigger allergic reactions, respiratory issues, or skin sensitivities.

It's essential to dilute essential oils properly, avoid ingesting them, and discontinue use if any adverse reactions occur. Pregnant individuals should also consult with healthcare providers before incorporating aromatherapy into their NVP management plan.

Acupressure and Acupuncture:

Acupressure and acupuncture are traditional Chinese medicine practices that involve applying pressure or inserting thin needles into specific points on the body to alleviate symptoms and restore balance.

While generally considered safe when performed by trained practitioners, there is limited scientific evidence supporting the efficacy and safety of acupressure and acupuncture for NVP.

Risks associated with acupressure and acupuncture may include bruising, discomfort at the insertion sites, and potential infections if proper hygiene protocols are not followed.

Mind-Body Interventions:

Mind-body interventions such as yoga, meditation, and relaxation techniques are generally safe and well-tolerated during pregnancy.

Pregnant individuals should practice mindfulness and yoga under the guidance of qualified instructors who are knowledgeable about the unique needs and limitations of pregnancy.

Modifications to poses and techniques may be necessary to accommodate the changing physiology and comfort levels of pregnant individuals.

Conclusion:

Safety considerations are paramount when incorporating non-pharmaceutical interventions (NPIs) into the management of nausea and vomiting in pregnancy (NVP). Pregnant individuals and healthcare providers must carefully assess the risks and benefits of NPIs, considering factors such as efficacy, safety profiles, and individual preferences. Open communication, informed decision-making, and collaboration between pregnant individuals and healthcare providers are essential for mitigating risks, optimizing maternal-fetal health, and ensuring positive pregnancy outcomes. It is imperative to prioritize safety and evidence-based care when implementing NPIs for NVP management, ultimately promoting the well-being of both the pregnant individual and the unborn child.

Monitoring and Adjusting Interventions Based on Individual Needs

Monitoring and adjusting interventions based on individual needs are crucial aspects of managing nausea and vomiting in pregnancy (NVP) effectively. In this chapter, we explore the importance of ongoing assessment, personalized care plans, and adaptive strategies to optimize outcomes for pregnant individuals experiencing NVP.

Ongoing Assessment:

Regular assessment of NVP symptoms, severity, and impact on daily functioning allows healthcare providers to monitor the progress of interventions and identify changes in symptoms over time.

Objective measures, such as frequency of vomiting episodes, severity of nausea on standardized scales, and changes in dietary intake, provide valuable data for tracking response to interventions.

Individualized Care Plans:

Tailoring interventions to the specific needs and preferences of each pregnant individual is essential for optimizing treatment outcomes and enhancing patient satisfaction.

Personalized care plans take into account factors such as symptom severity, gestational age, coexisting medical conditions, medication preferences, and lifestyle factors.

Flexibility in Treatment Approaches:

Recognizing that NVP symptoms can fluctuate throughout pregnancy, healthcare providers should remain flexible in their approach to intervention strategies.

Adjustments to treatment modalities, dosages, frequency of interventions, and complementary therapies may be necessary to address changing symptom patterns and evolving patient needs.

Patient Engagement and Collaboration:

Encouraging active participation and collaboration with pregnant individuals fosters a sense of empowerment, ownership, and trust in the therapeutic process.

Shared decision-making, open communication, and mutual respect between healthcare providers and patients are fundamental principles of patient-centered care.

Regular Follow-up:

Scheduled follow-up appointments allow healthcare providers to reassess NVP symptoms, evaluate treatment efficacy, address emerging concerns, and provide ongoing support and guidance.

Frequent communication between healthcare visits, through telemedicine, phone consultations, or secure messaging platforms, enables pregnant individuals to access timely guidance and support as needed.

Conclusion:

Monitoring and adjusting interventions based on individual needs are integral components of comprehensive care for nausea and vomiting in pregnancy (NVP). By embracing a patient-centered approach, healthcare providers can tailor interventions, engage in collaborative decision-making, and provide personalized support to pregnant individuals experiencing NVP. Through ongoing assessment, flexibility in treatment approaches, and regular follow-up, healthcare providers can optimize outcomes, enhance patient satisfaction, and promote the well-being of pregnant individuals throughout the course of pregnancy. It is essential to prioritize individualized care, adapt interventions as needed, and maintain open lines of communication to ensure the best possible outcomes for pregnant individuals experiencing NVP.

CHAPTER 8

INTEGRATIVE APPROACHES TO NVP MANAGEMENT

Integrative approaches to managing nausea and vomiting in pregnancy (NVP) involve combining various non-pharmaceutical interventions (NPIs) to address symptoms comprehensively while promoting overall well-being. In this chapter, we explore the principles, strategies, and benefits of integrating multiple NPIs for the effective management of NVP.

Holistic Perspective:

Integrative approaches to NVP management recognize the interconnectedness of physical, emotional, and psychological factors contributing to symptoms.

By adopting a holistic perspective, pregnant individuals and healthcare providers can explore diverse NPIs that address the multifaceted nature of NVP.

Multimodal Interventions:

Integrative NVP management involves combining multiple NPIs, such as dietary modifications, lifestyle changes, mind-body practices, and supportive therapies, to create a personalized care plan tailored to the individual's needs.

By integrating diverse interventions, pregnant individuals can access a range of tools and resources to alleviate symptoms and enhance overall quality of life.

Individualized Care:

Integrative approaches prioritize individualized care, taking into account the unique experiences, preferences, and circumstances of each pregnant individual.

Healthcare providers collaborate closely with pregnant individuals to co-create personalized NVP management plans that reflect their values, goals, and treatment preferences.

Comprehensive Support:

Integrative NVP management extends beyond symptom relief to encompass holistic support for physical, emotional, and social well-being.

In addition to addressing NVP symptoms, integrative approaches may include strategies for stress reduction, emotional support, nutritional counseling, and lifestyle optimization.

Collaboration and Coordination:

Effective integrative NVP management relies on collaboration and coordination among healthcare providers from various disciplines, including obstetrics, midwifery, nutrition, psychology, and complementary medicine.

By fostering interdisciplinary collaboration, healthcare teams can leverage diverse expertise and perspectives to deliver comprehensive, patient-centered care.

Conclusion:

Integrative approaches to managing nausea and vomiting in pregnancy (NVP) offer a holistic framework for addressing symptoms, enhancing well-being, and promoting optimal pregnancy outcomes. By integrating multiple non-pharmaceutical interventions (NPIs), adopting a personalized approach to care, and fostering collaboration among healthcare providers, pregnant individuals can access comprehensive support that aligns with their unique needs and preferences. Through an integrative lens, NVP management becomes not only about symptom control but also about empowering pregnant individuals to thrive physically, emotionally, and psychologically during this transformative time.

Combining Multiple NPIs for Enhanced Symptom Relief

Combining multiple non-pharmaceutical interventions (NPIs) offers a comprehensive approach to managing nausea and vomiting in pregnancy (NVP), enhancing symptom relief, and improving overall well-being. In this chapter, we explore the synergistic effects and practical strategies for integrating diverse NPIs to address the multifaceted nature of NVP.

Synergistic Effects:

Combining multiple NPIs capitalizes on the synergistic effects of different interventions, amplifying their individual benefits and enhancing overall symptom relief.

By targeting NVP symptoms through various pathways and mechanisms, combined NPIs can provide comprehensive relief and improve the effectiveness of treatment.

Tailored Treatment Plans:

Tailoring treatment plans to the individual needs and preferences of pregnant individuals is essential when combining multiple NPIs.

Healthcare providers collaborate closely with pregnant individuals to develop personalized care plans that integrate a combination of dietary modifications, lifestyle changes, complementary therapies, and supportive interventions.

Multimodal Approaches:

Multimodal approaches to NVP management involve combining NPIs from different categories, such as dietary modifications, physical activity, relaxation techniques, and psychological support.

Pregnant individuals may benefit from a combination of strategies that address physical symptoms, emotional well-being, and lifestyle factors contributing to NVP.

Sequential and Simultaneous Interventions:

Sequential interventions involve implementing NPIs in a stepwise manner, with adjustments made based on symptom response and individual needs.

Simultaneous interventions involve integrating multiple NPIs concurrently to address NVP symptoms comprehensively and provide immediate relief.

Monitoring and Adjustment:

Regular monitoring of NVP symptoms, treatment response, and side effects is essential when combining multiple NPIs.

Healthcare providers work collaboratively with pregnant individuals to assess the effectiveness of interventions, make necessary adjustments, and optimize treatment outcomes.

Conclusion:

Combining multiple non-pharmaceutical interventions (NPIs) offers a holistic and personalized approach to managing nausea and vomiting in pregnancy (NVP), enhancing symptom relief, and promoting overall well-being. By integrating diverse strategies, tailoring treatment plans to individual needs, and fostering collaboration between healthcare providers and pregnant individuals, combined NPIs can provide comprehensive support throughout pregnancy. Through a multifaceted approach, pregnant individuals can access a range of tools and resources to alleviate NVP symptoms, optimize pregnancy outcomes, and enhance their pregnancy experience.

Integrating NPIs with Pharmacological Interventions When Necessary

While non-pharmaceutical interventions (NPIs) serve as foundational approaches for managing nausea and vomiting in pregnancy (NVP), there are instances where pharmacological interventions may be necessary to alleviate severe symptoms and improve maternal well-being. In this chapter, we explore the principles, considerations, and practical strategies for integrating NPIs with pharmacological interventions when appropriate in the management of NVP.

131

Holistic Treatment Approach:

Integrating NPIs with pharmacological interventions reflects a holistic treatment approach that considers both non-pharmacological and pharmacological options based on the individual needs and preferences of pregnant individuals.

By combining multiple treatment modalities, healthcare providers can address NVP symptoms comprehensively while minimizing risks and optimizing treatment outcomes.

Individualized Care Plans:

Individualized care plans are essential when integrating NPIs with pharmacological interventions, taking into account the severity of NVP symptoms, maternal health status, fetal considerations, and treatment preferences.

Pregnant individuals and healthcare providers collaborate closely to develop personalized treatment plans that balance the benefits and risks of both non-pharmacological and pharmacological interventions.

Targeted Symptom Relief:

NPIs may serve as adjunctive therapies to pharmacological interventions, enhancing their effectiveness and promoting symptom relief.

Integrating NPIs such as dietary modifications, lifestyle changes, relaxation techniques, and complementary therapies can help manage NVP symptoms and reduce the reliance on pharmacological agents.

Minimizing Risks:

When integrating NPIs with pharmacological interventions, healthcare providers prioritize minimizing risks and adverse effects associated with medication use during pregnancy.

Close monitoring, careful selection of medications, adherence to recommended dosages, and regular follow-up appointments are essential for ensuring maternal and fetal safety.

Shared Decision-Making:

Shared decision-making between pregnant individuals and healthcare providers is central to the integration of NPIs with pharmacological interventions.

Open communication, informed consent, and collaborative discussions empower pregnant individuals to actively participate in treatment decisions, voice their concerns, and express their treatment preferences.

Conclusion:

Integrating non-pharmaceutical interventions (NPIs) with pharmacological interventions when necessary offers a balanced and individualized approach to managing nausea and vomiting in pregnancy (NVP). By combining multiple treatment modalities, healthcare providers can address NVP symptoms comprehensively while prioritizing maternal and fetal safety. Through shared decision-making and personalized care planning, pregnant individuals can access a range of treatment options that align with their values, goals, and preferences, ultimately enhancing their pregnancy experience and promoting optimal outcomes for both mother and baby.

Holistic Approaches to Promoting Overall Maternal Well-being

Holistic approaches to promoting overall maternal well-being recognize the interconnectedness of physical, emotional, and social factors that influence the pregnancy experience. In this chapter, we explore the principles, strategies, and benefits of holistic care in managing nausea and vomiting in pregnancy (NVP) while supporting the broader health and wellness of pregnant individuals.

Comprehensive Assessment:

Holistic care begins with a comprehensive assessment of the pregnant individual's physical health, emotional well-being, lifestyle factors, and social support networks.

Healthcare providers take a holistic approach to understanding the individual's unique needs, preferences, and challenges related to NVP and pregnancy.

Multifaceted Support:

Holistic approaches to NVP management encompass a range of non-pharmaceutical interventions (NPIs), including dietary modifications, lifestyle changes, complementary therapies, stress reduction techniques, and emotional support.

By addressing NVP symptoms and promoting overall well-being through multiple avenues, holistic care aims to optimize maternal health and pregnancy outcomes.

Individualized Care Plans:

Holistic care plans are tailored to the specific needs, preferences, and circumstances of each pregnant individual.

Healthcare providers collaborate closely with pregnant individuals to co-create personalized care plans that integrate a combination of NPIs and address the holistic dimensions of health and wellness.

Emphasis on Self-care:

Holistic approaches prioritize self-care practices that empower pregnant individuals to take an active role in promoting their own health and well-being.

Self-care strategies may include mindfulness practices, relaxation techniques, physical activity, nutrition education, and stress management skills.

Integration of Support Networks:

Holistic care extends beyond the clinical setting to integrate support networks, community resources, and peer support groups.

Pregnant individuals are encouraged to connect with social networks, online communities, and support groups where they can share experiences, seek advice, and access emotional support.

Continuity of Care:

Holistic care emphasizes continuity of care throughout the prenatal journey, from early pregnancy to postpartum recovery.

Healthcare providers offer ongoing support, monitoring, and guidance to pregnant individuals, ensuring that their holistic needs are addressed at every stage of pregnancy and beyond.

Conclusion:

Holistic approaches to promoting overall maternal well-being offer pregnant individuals comprehensive support for managing nausea and vomiting in pregnancy (NVP) while fostering physical, emotional, and social health. By integrating diverse non-pharmaceutical interventions, emphasizing self-care practices, and fostering collaboration between healthcare providers and pregnant individuals, holistic care aims to optimize pregnancy outcomes and enhance the pregnancy experience. Through a holistic lens, NVP management becomes not only about symptom control but also about empowering pregnant individuals to thrive physically, emotionally, and socially during this transformative time.

CHAPTER 9

FUTURE DIRECTIONS AND RESEARCH OPPORTUNITIES

As our understanding of nausea and vomiting in pregnancy (NVP) continues to evolve, there are numerous opportunities for future research to advance the field of non-pharmaceutical interventions (NPIs) and enhance the care provided to pregnant individuals. In this chapter, we explore potential future directions and research opportunities that can further optimize NVP management and improve pregnancy outcomes.

Mechanistic Studies:

Investigating the underlying mechanisms of NVP can provide valuable insights into the pathophysiology of the condition and identify novel targets for intervention.

Future research may focus on elucidating the neurophysiological, hormonal, and gastrointestinal factors contributing to NVP to inform the development of targeted therapies.

Comparative Effectiveness Research:

Comparative effectiveness research involves evaluating the relative efficacy, safety, and cost-effectiveness of different NPIs for managing NVP.

Comparative studies can help identify the most effective interventions for specific subgroups of pregnant individuals and inform evidence-based treatment guidelines.

Longitudinal Studies:

Longitudinal studies that follow pregnant individuals from early pregnancy through the postpartum period can provide insights into the natural history of NVP, treatment trajectories, and long-term outcomes.

By tracking NVP symptoms, treatment responses, and maternal-fetal outcomes over time, longitudinal research can inform personalized care approaches and identify predictors of treatment success.

Patient-Centered Outcomes Research:

Patient-centered outcomes research focuses on outcomes that matter most to pregnant individuals, such as symptom relief, quality of life, functional status, and treatment satisfaction.

Future studies should prioritize patient-reported outcomes and incorporate pregnant individuals' perspectives, preferences, and values into research design and outcome assessment.

Implementation Science:

Implementation science aims to bridge the gap between research evidence and clinical practice by identifying strategies to effectively translate NVP management guidelines into real-world settings.

Research on implementation strategies, barriers, and facilitators can help optimize the delivery of NPIs in diverse healthcare settings and improve access to evidence-based care.

Novel Interventions:

Exploring novel NPIs, such as digital health interventions, wearable devices, mobile applications, and telehealth platforms, can expand the range of options available for NVP management.

Future research may investigate the feasibility, acceptability, and effectiveness of innovative interventions that leverage technology to support pregnant individuals and enhance symptom management.

Conclusion:

Future directions and research opportunities in the field of non-pharmaceutical interventions for nausea and vomiting in pregnancy (NVP) hold great promise for improving the care and outcomes of pregnant individuals. By advancing mechanistic understanding, conducting comparative effectiveness research, embracing patient-centered approaches, and exploring novel interventions, researchers can address key gaps in knowledge and enhance the evidence base for NVP management. Collaborative efforts across disciplines, innovative research methodologies, and a commitment to patient-centered care are essential for realizing the full potential of non-pharmaceutical interventions in optimizing pregnancy health and well-being.

Emerging Trends in NPIs for NVP Management

As our understanding of nausea and vomiting in pregnancy (NVP) evolves, emerging trends in non-pharmaceutical interventions (NPIs) offer new avenues for managing symptoms and promoting maternal well-being. In this chapter, we explore cutting-edge approaches, innovative technologies, and evolving strategies that are shaping the landscape of NVP management.

Digital Health Interventions:

Digital health interventions, including mobile applications, wearable devices, and online platforms, offer novel solutions for managing NVP symptoms and supporting pregnant individuals remotely.

Mobile apps can provide symptom tracking, personalized recommendations, educational resources, and virtual support networks to help pregnant individuals navigate NVP more effectively.

Telemedicine and Virtual Care:

Telemedicine and virtual care platforms enable pregnant individuals to access healthcare services, consultations, and support remotely, reducing barriers to care and increasing accessibility.

Telemedicine appointments allow healthcare providers to conduct virtual assessments, monitor symptoms, and deliver personalized recommendations for NVP management from a distance.

Personalized Medicine Approaches:

Personalized medicine approaches leverage genetic, hormonal, and physiological factors to tailor NVP management strategies to the individual's unique characteristics and needs.

Genetic profiling, biomarker analysis, and hormone testing may help identify predictors of NVP severity, treatment response, and susceptibility to specific interventions.

Mind-Body Interventions:

Mind-body interventions, such as mindfulness-based stress reduction

(MBSR), yoga, meditation, and relaxation techniques, are gaining recognition for their potential to alleviate NVP symptoms and improve maternal well-being.

Integrating mind-body practices into NVP management plans can help pregnant individuals cultivate resilience, reduce stress, and cope more effectively with NVP-related discomfort.

Complementary and Integrative Therapies:

Complementary and integrative therapies, including acupuncture, acupressure, herbal remedies, and aromatherapy, are emerging as promising adjunctive treatments for NVP management.

Integrating evidence-based complementary therapies into conventional care approaches may offer additional options for symptom relief and enhance the holistic care of pregnant individuals.

Lifestyle Modifications:

Lifestyle modifications, such as dietary changes, hydration strategies, sleep hygiene practices, and physical activity

145

recommendations, remain foundational components of NVP management.

Emerging trends focus on optimizing lifestyle factors to support overall maternal health, enhance symptom management, and improve pregnancy outcomes.

Conclusion:

Emerging trends in non-pharmaceutical interventions (NPIs) for nausea and vomiting in pregnancy (NVP) reflect ongoing innovation, integration of technology, and a growing emphasis on personalized, holistic care approaches. By embracing digital health interventions, telemedicine platforms, personalized medicine approaches, mind-body interventions, complementary therapies, and lifestyle modifications, healthcare providers can offer pregnant individuals a diverse array of options for managing NVP symptoms and promoting maternal well-being. Continued research, collaboration, and innovation are essential for advancing NVP management and improving pregnancy outcomes in the evolving landscape of maternal healthcare.

Areas for Further Research and Innovation

As the field of non-pharmaceutical interventions (NPIs) for nausea and vomiting in pregnancy (NVP) continues to evolve, there are several areas ripe for further research and innovation. In this chapter, we explore key domains where advancements in research and innovation hold the potential to enhance NVP management and improve the pregnancy experience for affected individuals.

Mechanistic Understanding:

Further research is needed to elucidate the underlying mechanisms driving NVP, including hormonal, neurophysiological, and gastrointestinal factors.

Investigating the molecular pathways and physiological processes involved in NVP can inform the development of targeted interventions and personalized treatment approaches.

Personalized Medicine:

There is a growing recognition of the heterogeneity of NVP presentations and responses to treatment among pregnant individuals.

Research focused on identifying biomarkers, genetic predispositions, and phenotypic characteristics associated with NVP can facilitate the delivery of personalized medicine and tailored interventions.

Digital Health Solutions:

Emerging technologies, such as mobile applications, wearable devices, and telehealth platforms, offer innovative opportunities for NVP management.

Future research may explore the feasibility and effectiveness of digital health solutions in delivering personalized support, symptom tracking, remote monitoring, and behavioral interventions for pregnant individuals experiencing NVP.

Psychosocial Factors:

Psychosocial factors, including stress, anxiety, depression, social support, and coping mechanisms, play a significant role in the experience and management of NVP.

Research aimed at understanding the interplay between psychosocial factors and

NVP can inform holistic approaches to care and interventions targeting mental health and well-being during pregnancy.

Complementary and Integrative Therapies:

Complementary and integrative therapies, such as acupuncture, acupressure, herbal remedies, and mindfulness practices, have shown promise in managing NVP symptoms.

Further research is warranted to evaluate the efficacy, safety, and mechanisms of action of these therapies, as well as their integration into mainstream healthcare settings.

Long-term Outcomes:

There is a need for longitudinal studies examining the long-term effects of NVP on maternal and child health outcomes beyond the perinatal period.

Research investigating the impact of NVP on maternal nutritional status, fetal development, birth outcomes, and postpartum health can provide valuable insights into the broader health implications of NVP.

Conclusion:

The pursuit of further research and innovation in non-pharmaceutical interventions for nausea and vomiting in pregnancy (NVP) holds great promise for improving the care and outcomes of affected individuals. By advancing mechanistic understanding, embracing personalized medicine, harnessing digital health solutions, addressing psychosocial factors, exploring complementary therapies, and investigating long-term outcomes, researchers can contribute to the development of evidence-based strategies that optimize NVP management and enhance the pregnancy experience. Collaborative efforts across disciplines, innovative research methodologies, and a commitment to patient-centered care are essential for advancing the field and addressing the evolving needs of pregnant individuals experiencing NVP.

Potential Implications for Clinical Practice and Public Health Policy

Understanding the potential implications of non-pharmaceutical interventions (NPIs) for

150

nausea and vomiting in pregnancy (NVP) on clinical practice and public health policy is essential for improving the care and outcomes of pregnant individuals. In this chapter, we explore the implications of NPIs for NVP management on both clinical practice and public health policy.

Clinical Practice Implications:

a. Personalized Care: NPIs offer opportunities for personalized care tailored to the individual needs and preferences of pregnant individuals experiencing NVP.

b. Multidisciplinary Approach: Implementing NPIs may require a multidisciplinary approach involving obstetricians, midwives, dietitians, psychologists, and other healthcare providers to address the multifaceted nature of NVP.

c. Shared Decision-Making: NPIs promote shared decision-making between healthcare providers and pregnant individuals, empowering patients to actively participate in their care and treatment decisions.

151

d. Continuity of Care: NPIs emphasize continuity of care throughout the prenatal period, ensuring that pregnant individuals receive consistent support and monitoring for NVP symptoms.

Public Health Policy Implications:

a. Education and Awareness: Public health policies should prioritize education and awareness initiatives to increase understanding of NVP among healthcare providers, pregnant individuals, and the general public.

b. Access to Care: Policies should aim to improve access to NVP management services, including NPIs, across diverse healthcare settings and communities.

c. Research Funding: Public health policy should support funding for research into the efficacy, safety, and cost-effectiveness of NPIs for NVP management, as well as their impact on maternal and child health outcomes.

d. Integration into Guidelines: Guidelines and protocols for NVP management should incorporate evidence-based recommendations for NPIs, ensuring that pregnant individuals receive comprehensive care aligned with best practices.

Conclusion:

The implications of non-pharmaceutical interventions for nausea and vomiting in pregnancy (NVP) on clinical practice and public health policy are profound, offering opportunities to improve care delivery, enhance patient outcomes, and promote maternal and child health. By embracing personalized care approaches, fostering multidisciplinary collaboration, promoting shared decision-making, and prioritizing education and research, healthcare systems and public health authorities can address the complex challenges of NVP management and improve the pregnancy experience for affected individuals. Moving forward, continued efforts to integrate NPIs into clinical practice guidelines and public health initiatives will be essential for advancing the field and optimizing outcomes for pregnant individuals experiencing NVP.

CHAPTER 10

CONCLUSION

In conclusion, the management of nausea and vomiting in pregnancy (NVP) presents a multifaceted challenge that requires a comprehensive and individualized approach. Non-pharmaceutical interventions (NPIs) play a crucial role in alleviating symptoms, promoting maternal well-being, and optimizing pregnancy outcomes for affected individuals. Throughout this book, we have explored various aspects of NPIs for NVP management, including their definition, significance, effectiveness, safety considerations, and integration into clinical practice and public health policy.

From dietary modifications and lifestyle changes to complementary therapies and psychosocial support, NPIs offer a diverse array of strategies to address the complex nature of NVP. By adopting a holistic perspective and embracing personalized care approaches, healthcare providers can empower pregnant individuals to actively participate in their treatment decisions and optimize their pregnancy experience.

154

Looking ahead, there are numerous opportunities for further research, innovation, and collaboration in the field of NVP management. Emerging trends, such as digital health solutions, personalized medicine, and integrative approaches, hold promise for advancing the care provided to pregnant individuals experiencing NVP. Moreover, ongoing efforts to integrate NPIs into clinical practice guidelines and public health initiatives will be essential for ensuring equitable access to evidence-based care and improving outcomes for pregnant individuals worldwide.

As we continue to expand our understanding of NVP and refine our approaches to management, it is imperative that we prioritize the needs, preferences, and experiences of pregnant individuals. By fostering a supportive and patient-centered approach to care, we can enhance the well-being of pregnant individuals, promote positive pregnancy experiences, and ultimately improve maternal and child health outcomes.

In closing, the journey to effectively manage nausea and vomiting in pregnancy requires collaboration, innovation, and a commitment to holistic care. Through continued research, education, and advocacy, we can strive to provide compassionate and evidence-based support to pregnant individuals experiencing NVP, ultimately enriching the journey of pregnancy and childbirth for all.

Summary of Key Findings and Insights:

"Non-Pharmaceutical Interventions for Nausea and Vomiting in Pregnancy" delves into the multifaceted aspects of managing nausea and vomiting in pregnancy (NVP) through non-pharmaceutical means. Here are the key findings and insights derived from the book:

Definition and Significance:

NVP is a common condition during pregnancy, characterized by nausea and vomiting that can significantly impact maternal quality of life and well-being.

Non-pharmaceutical interventions offer safe and effective alternatives to pharmacological treatments for managing NVP.

Understanding NVP:

NVP is a complex condition influenced by hormonal changes, gastrointestinal factors, and psychosocial stressors.

Effective management of NVP requires a holistic understanding of its underlying mechanisms and contributing factors.

Causes and Contributing Factors:

Various factors contribute to the development and severity of NVP, including hormonal fluctuations, dietary triggers, psychological stress, and genetic predispositions.

Impact on Maternal Health:

NVP can have significant implications for maternal health, leading to dehydration, malnutrition, electrolyte imbalances, and psychological distress.

Addressing NVP symptoms is crucial for promoting maternal well-being and ensuring optimal pregnancy outcomes.

Non-Pharmaceutical Interventions (NPIs):

NPIs encompass a wide range of strategies, including dietary modifications, lifestyle changes, complementary therapies, and psychosocial support.

Integrating NPIs into NVP management can alleviate symptoms, improve maternal comfort, and enhance overall pregnancy experiences.

Safety and Effectiveness:

NPIs offer safe and effective alternatives to pharmacological interventions for managing NVP, with minimal risk of adverse effects for both the pregnant individual and the fetus.

Evidence-based practices and guidelines help healthcare providers select appropriate NPIs tailored to individual needs and preferences.

Holistic Approaches:

Holistic approaches to NVP management recognize the interconnectedness of physical, emotional, and social factors influencing the pregnancy experience.

Integrating diverse NPIs and promoting self-care practices contribute to holistic care and improved maternal well-being.

Future Directions and Research Opportunities:

Future research directions include mechanistic studies, personalized medicine approaches, digital health solutions, and long-term outcome assessments.

Collaborative efforts across disciplines and innovative research methodologies are essential for advancing the field of NVP management.

Addressing Multifaceted Factors:

NVP is a complex condition influenced by various factors including hormonal changes, dietary triggers, psychological stress, and individual differences in physiology. A holistic approach acknowledges the interplay of these factors and seeks to address them comprehensively rather than focusing solely on symptom management.

Promoting Overall Well-being:

Pregnancy is a transformative journey that

159

encompasses physical, emotional, and social dimensions of health. A holistic approach to NVP management recognizes the importance of promoting overall maternal well-being beyond just alleviating nausea and vomiting symptoms. It considers the impact of NVP on maternal quality of life, nutritional status, emotional health, and functional capacity.

Tailoring Care to Individual Needs:
Every pregnant individual experiences NVP differently, with unique symptoms, triggers, and preferences for treatment. A holistic approach allows healthcare providers to tailor care plans to meet the specific needs and preferences of each individual. By considering the whole person, including their cultural background, lifestyle factors, and personal beliefs, healthcare providers can develop personalized strategies that resonate with the pregnant individual.

Integrating Multiple Modalities:
Holistic approaches to NVP management integrate a diverse range of non-pharmaceutical interventions such as dietary modifications, lifestyle changes,

complementary therapies, stress reduction techniques, and psychosocial support. By combining multiple modalities, healthcare providers can offer pregnant individuals a comprehensive toolkit to manage NVP effectively.

Empowering Pregnant Individuals:

A holistic approach empowers pregnant individuals to take an active role in their own care and decision-making process. By providing education, resources, and support, healthcare providers enable pregnant individuals to make informed choices that align with their values and preferences. This empowerment fosters a sense of autonomy and self-efficacy, which are essential components of holistic care.

Considering Long-term Implications:

Pregnancy is a dynamic process that extends beyond the immediate experience of NVP. A holistic approach considers the long-term implications of NVP on maternal and fetal health outcomes, including nutritional status, birth outcomes, and postpartum recovery. By addressing NVP comprehensively, healthcare providers can mitigate potential long-term consequences and optimize overall pregnancy outcomes.

Final Thoughts on the Future of NPIs in Improving Maternal and Fetal Health

As we conclude our exploration of non-pharmaceutical interventions (NPIs) for nausea and vomiting in pregnancy (NVP) in the book titled "Non-Pharmaceutical Interventions for Nausea and Vomiting in Pregnancy," it's evident that the future holds promising opportunities for enhancing maternal and fetal health outcomes. Here are some final thoughts on the future of NPIs in improving maternal and fetal health:

Personalized Care: The future of NPIs lies in personalized care approaches that consider the unique needs, preferences, and circumstances of each pregnant individual. By tailoring interventions to individual characteristics and responses, healthcare providers can optimize the effectiveness of NVP management strategies.

Integrative Approaches: Integrating NPIs with conventional medical care offers a holistic approach to NVP management that addresses the multifaceted nature of the condition. By combining dietary modifications, lifestyle changes, complementary therapies, and psychosocial support, healthcare providers can provide comprehensive care that promotes maternal well-being and fetal health.

Evidence-Based Practice: The future of NPIs depends on continued research and evidence-based practice. Rigorous studies are needed to evaluate the safety, efficacy, and cost-effectiveness of NPIs in managing NVP and improving pregnancy outcomes. By generating high-quality evidence, healthcare providers can make informed decisions and optimize care delivery.

Patient-Centered Care: Central to the future of NPIs is the principle of patient-centered care. Pregnant individuals should be actively engaged in their care and empowered to make informed decisions about NVP management. By fostering open communication, mutual respect, and shared decision-making, healthcare providers can build trusting relationships and enhance patient outcomes.

Collaborative Efforts:

Improving maternal and fetal health outcomes requires collaborative efforts across disciplines, healthcare settings, and communities. By fostering partnerships between healthcare providers, researchers, policymakers, and community stakeholders, we can develop innovative strategies, share best practices, and address systemic barriers to care.

Advocacy and Education:

Advocating for the importance of NVP management and raising awareness about the availability of NPIs are essential for improving maternal and fetal health outcomes. Education initiatives aimed at healthcare providers, pregnant individuals, and the broader community can dispel myths, reduce stigma, and promote access to evidence-based care.